Therapeutic Claims
in Multiple Sclerosis

SECOND EDITION

William A. Sibley, M.D.

Department of Neurology
University of Arizona
Tucson, AZ

and the

Therapeutic Claims Committee
of the International Federation
of Multiple Sclerosis Societies

Demos Publications, 156 Fifth Avenue, New York, New York 10010

Made in the United States of America

This book is written for informational purposes only. Nothing contained in it should be interpreted as a recommended treatment for any individual patient; such a decision can only be made by the patient's physician who can consider merits, risks, past history, associated illnesses, and many other factors. The opinions expressed about the general usefulness, or lack of usefulness, of various therapies are those of the Therapeutic Claims Committee of the International Federation of Multiple Sclerosis Societies (IFMSS) and are based on information available from a variety of sources, published and unpublished, and collective personal experience.

Great care has been taken to maintain the accuracy of the information contained in this volume. However, Demos Publications and the IFMSS cannot be held responsible for errors or for any consequences arising from the use of the information contained herein.

ISBN: 0-939-957-16-7
ISBN: 0-939-957-13-2 (paperback)

LC: 88-071343

IFMSS Therapeutic Claims Committee

William Austin Sibley, *Chairman*
Professor of Neurology
University of Arizona
Chairman, Subcommittee on Therapeutic Claims

Helmut J. Bauer
Professor of Neurology, Emeritus
University of Gottingen
Vice-Chairman, Medical Advisory Board, IFMSS

Kenneth P. Johnson
Professor and Chairman of Neurology
University of Maryland

Reginald E. Kelly
Physician and Dean Emeritus
Institute of Neurology
Queen Square, London
Chairman, Medical Advisory Board, IFMSS

W. Ian McDonald
Professor, University Department
of Clinical Neurology
The National Hospital, Queen Square, London

William J. McIlroy
Associate Professor of Neurology
University of Toronto
National Medical Advisor, MS Society of Canada
Chairman-Elect, Medical Advisory Board, IFMSS

Donald W. Paty
Professor and Chairman of Neurology
University of British Columbia
Secretary, Medical Advisory Board, IFMSS

Olivier Sabouraud
Professor and Chairman of Neurology
University of Rennes Medical Center

Labe C. Scheinberg
Professor of Neurology and Rehabilitation Medicine
Albert Einstein College of Medicine

Stanley van den Noort
Professor of Neurology
California College of Medicine
Past-Chairman, Medical Advisory Board
National MS Society, U.S.A.

PREFACE

Since publication of the first edition of *Therapeutic Claims in Multiple Sclerosis,* there have been numerous trials of treatment conducted in many countries in an effort to find an effective therapy for MS. Several of these treatments have been reported to have a positive effect in reducing the frequency of attacks or in slowing progression in well-designed studies. Examples include plasmapheresis, alpha- and beta-interferon, copolymer I, total lymphoid irradiation, and cyclophosphamide. Nevertheless, there are still conflicting reports about these and other therapies.

There are several new members of the Therapeutic Claims Committee, and all members are actively treating patients with MS on a daily basis. All have participated, or are participating in, active trials of therapy with various agents. They have used most, if not all, of the treatment methods seriously advocated during the past two decades. As Chairman of the Committee, I have conducted a poll of the members about their current practices, and the results are summarized in this volume.

All experienced neurologists agree that, in spite of certain encouraging signs, much more effective treatment is necessary—both for the acute attack of MS and for progressively worsening MS.

Although the exact cause of MS remains unknown, encouraging progress has been made in understanding triggering factors, and one may hope that this will result in more effective preventive measures.

One of the most exciting developments in recent years has been a dramatic improvement in ability to measure the activity and progress of MS, and magnetic resonance imaging has been responsible for this. Since the essence of research is accurate measurement, it seems likely that progress will be more rapid in the next few years.

This new edition summarizes these new developments. In addition, the general management and symptomatic treatment recommendations prepared with the advice of the Medical Management Committee of the IFMSS, chaired by Dr. Donald Paty, are reported in Chapter 5. Some of the descriptions of old treatments have been shortened or eliminated, in order to keep the book approximately the same size.

The Committee remains indebted to Dr. Joe R. Brown, a former member chiefly responsible for writing the first edition. We wish also to express special gratitude to Dr. Byron Waksman, Vice President for Research and Medical Programs, National Multiple Sclerosis Society, U.S.A., who has provided invaluable assistance as research consultant in reading and correcting the manuscript. He has also expertly handled the many important details necessary to bring the volume to publication.

W. A. Sibley
Chairman, Board of Editors

CONTENTS

Introduction

Multiple sclerosis (MS) is primarily a disease of the central nervous system (CNS)—the brain and spinal cord. Before proceeding to a discussion of MS, a brief review of the CNS is appropriate.

THE CENTRAL NERVOUS SYSTEM

The CNS consists of the brain (cerebrum, cerebellum, and brainstem), the spinal cord and optic nerves (Fig. 1-1), and is composed of gray and white matter.

In the CNS there are four kinds of cells: nerve cells, oligodendroglia, astrocytes, and microglia. These cells are fed by nutrients that are carried to the CNS by the blood through blood vessels (arteries, capillaries, and veins).

The nerve cells are the main component of gray matter. Each nerve cell has a *nerve fiber (axon),* which connects the cell body with the muscles, the sensory organs such as the eyes, ears, and skin, or the viscera such as the heart and stomach. The nerve cells and their fibers are responsible for sending messages back and forth within the CNS and between the CNS and the rest of the body. Some nerve fibers are short, running between adjacent nerve cells. The longest fibers run the full length of the spinal cord and may be several feet in length.

Individual nerve fibers are wrapped in numerous thin layers

1

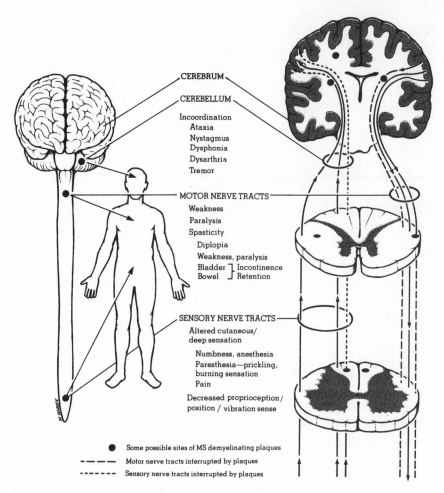

CEREBRUM

CEREBELLUM
Incoordination
 Ataxia
 Nystagmus
 Dysphonia
 Dysarthria
 Tremor

MOTOR NERVE TRACTS
Weakness
Paralysis
Spasticity
 Diplopia
 Weakness, paralysis
 Bladder ⎤ Incontinence
 Bowel ⎦ Retention

SENSORY NERVE TRACTS
Altered cutaneous/
deep sensation
 Numbness, anesthesia
 Paresthesia—prickling,
 burning sensation
 Pain
 Decreased proprioception/
 position / vibration sense

●   Some possible sites of MS demyelinating plaques
– – – – Motor nerve tracts interrupted by plaques
- - - - - - Sensory nerve tracts interrupted by plaques

FIG. 1-1. Diagram of the CNS, including all the principal regions in which MS lesions appear.

of a substance called *myelin,* which acts as an insulator and speeds the transmission of messages along the nerve fiber (Fig. 1-2). Myelin is composed of fats and proteins, and it is myelin that gives a creamy white color to the white matter. Myelin is produced and maintained by the oligodendroglia. These cells send out many branches, which end in expanded sheets that wrap around the nerve fibers and form the myelin.

Astrocytes also sprout branching processes, which support

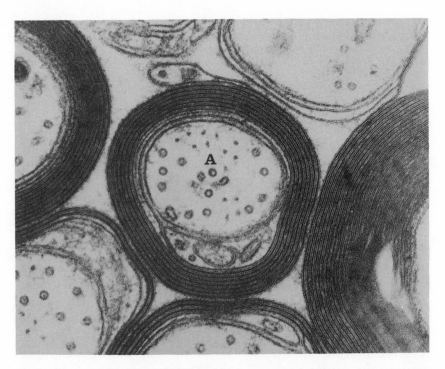

FIG. 1-2. Electronmicrograph shows several normal myelin sheaths at high magnification. Each sheath is seen as the spirally wrapped membrane around a nerve fiber or axon (A). (x 38,500.)

other structures in the CNS. They also control, in a way not yet fully understood, the passage of soluble substances between the blood vessels and the other CNS cells. This control is called the *blood–brain barrier*. Ordinarily, there is limited movement of substances through the walls of the blood vessels into the CNS. Just as the blood brings nutrients and removes waste products, it may also bring substances that cause harm, especially if such substances can pass the blood–brain barrier.

Whenever there is damage to the CNS, it is the job of the microglia to remove debris. After this clean-up, the astrocytes, whose job it is to maintain the structural integrity of the CNS, complete the healing process by producing a scar, which fills the damaged area in the same way a fibrous scar develops after a cut in the skin.

WHAT IS MULTIPLE SCLEROSIS?

Multiple sclerosis is an inflammatory disease of the CNS (brain, spinal cord, and optic nerves), characterized by the occurrence of random patches of inflammation, with loss of myelin (the insulation surrounding nerve fibers in the white matter of the brain and spinal cord). The patches, or "plaques," occur sporadically; the number of plaques and the frequency of new ones vary widely from person to person. Some patients have only a few, but in others there are many. The plaques may become scars, and the name "multiple sclerosis" refers to the multiple scars that develop in the CNS (Fig. 1-3).

During days or weeks after development of a new plaque, nerve impulse conduction through the area is abnormal, being either slower or blocked: symptoms of trouble are then at their maximum. This is variously called an *"exacerbation," "attack," "bout,"* or *"relapse."* Later, as inflammation in the new plaque subsides, nerve impulse conduction improves, but at a reduced speed (because of loss of the myelin insulation): at that time symptoms improve (remission). It is of little immediate importance to the person with MS that the nerve impulse reaches its target a few thousandths of a second more slowly than normal; but such abnormal conduction is insecure, contributes to the more rapid fatigability of MS patients, and further slowing or failure of conduction may occur temporarily with fever or exertion. This explains why symptoms may fluctuate in severity from hour to hour.

Sometimes damage to the nerve fibers is irreparable and the ability to conduct impulses is lost. Symptoms then become permanent.

THE DIAGNOSIS OF MULTIPLE SCLEROSIS: HOW ARE THE PLAQUES DETECTED?

MS may produce a variety of symptoms, and characteristic ones cause suspicion of the disease in the mind of an experienced physician. Symptoms usually last for days or weeks before improving; the most common time for improvement is 4–12 weeks

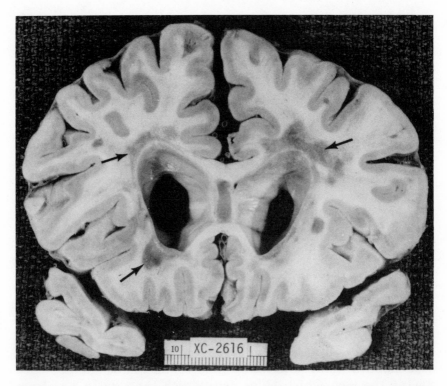

FIG. 1-3. A slice of the brain from a patient with MS shows many large MS plaques (arrows), which appear as gray areas in the white matter. It is the fatty substances in the myelin that make this matter white. The plaques are glassy in appearance and gray, due to the loss of the myelin and to scarring.

after onset. At least two-thirds of patients, in the beginning, have symptoms that come and go; in another 15% of patients, symptoms are slowly progressive from onset, and remissions never occur.

Common symptoms include dimness of vision in one or both eyes, weakness of one or both legs, numbness and tingling (paresthesias) in the face, arms, legs, and over the trunk. Often there is a "band-like" numbness around the chest or abdomen. Frequently, paresthesias are provoked by flexion (forward bending) of the neck. Vertigo, double vision, slurred speech, and urinary urgency or incontinence are also frequent symptoms. A feeling of severe fatigue is common in MS, especially when the illness is active.

These symptoms are usually associated with *objective changes on neurological examination (Fig. 1-4)*. Symptoms alone are never adequate to warrant a diagnosis of MS. The diagnosis must be made by a neurologist or other physician thoroughly familiar with the many other diseases of the nervous system. A clear distinction must be made between these ailments and MS. The diagnosis is often difficult and must rest primarily on medical judgment rather than on any single laboratory test.

In addition to the neurological history and examination, there are other aids to diagnosis. The most important of these is the *magnetic resonance imaging (MRI) scanner*. The MRI scan reveals many abnormal areas that are invisible on the older computer tomography (CT) scan. Some of these abnormal areas (lesions) are plaques of demyelination, and some represent inflamed areas of tissue that may not be seen on repeat scans. Using a large electromagnet, a radiofrequency stimulator, and a computer, this remarkable new diagnostic tool now enables us to visualize and count the number of lesions (Fig. 1-5 and 1-6).

A chemical compound called gadolinium can be administered during the test, which helps distinguish the new lesions from the old. Repeat scans also make it possible to verify the occurrence of new areas of abnormality. A completely effective treatment for MS would totally prevent the occurrence of new lesions seen on the MRI, but would not remove old scars.

Good as it is, however, the MRI scan is not infallible. Although it is positive in approximately 90% of patients, it is not positive in all, if one uses diagnostic criteria that were found to be reliable before the introduction of this new scanning technique. Some of the plaques in the spinal cord, brainstem, and optic nerves are still missed by MRI; evoked response testing (see below) can be used to detect these. The MRI scan alone cannot be used to diagnose MS because similar appearances can be seen in a number of other diseases.

In many patients there are also characteristic *changes in the spinal fluid* that aid diagnosis. These changes consist of an increase in the white blood cell content in some cases, and an increase (or change in the character) of immunoglobulins and

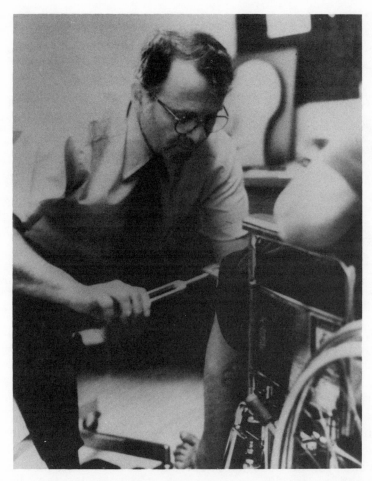

FIG. 1-4. The neurological examination is the single most important element in the diagnosis of MS. The use of a "reflex hammer" to test reflexes, illustrated here, is particularly useful in demonstrating increased reflexes (hyperreflexia) and even spasticity (described on p. 93) in the presence of weakness, a common and important finding in patients with MS.

other substances in the spinal fluid. Although these changes are not a specific test for MS, they are helpful in diagnosis when considered by the physician in conjunction with the history and examination. A lumbar puncture (spinal tap) therefore remains important in many cases for diagnosis, and in many other cases

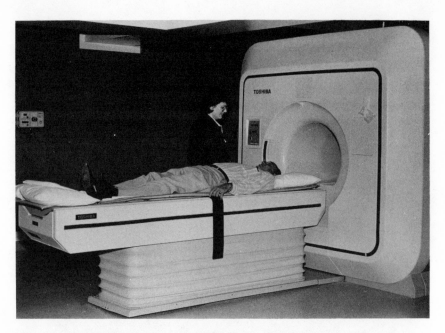

FIG. 1-5. Patient preparing to enter an MRI scanner. There are no x-rays involved. MRI is many times more sensitive in detecting the lesions of MS than the older CT scanner.

for research purposes: for example, to determine the effect of "treatment X" on the spinal fluid.

There are other *electrodiagnostic tests* that measure the rate of nerve impulse conduction through various portions of the nervous system. Conduction rates are usually quite slow in the nerve fibers as they pass through the demyelinated plaques. Thus, the visual evoked potential (VEP) test (also called the visual evoked response: VER) measures the rate of conduction between the retina and the occipital lobe (visual area) of the brain; it is especially reliable in confirming unsuspected plaques in the optic nerves, which may not be detected in any other way (Fig. 1-7). The auditory evoked potential test is used in a similar manner to detect lesions in the brainstem, which may not be seen by MRI. Sensory evoked responses can also measure conduction velocities in nerve tracts carrying touch and pain sensation to the brain.

There is *no established blood test* for MS at this time.

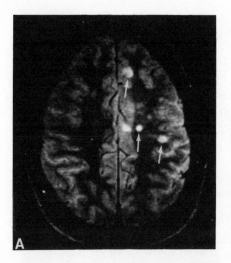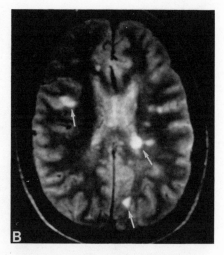

FIG. 1-6. Two MRI scan "slices" show abnormal areas (lesions) in the brain of a 28-year-old woman with MS, who has minimal weakness of the right arm and leg. In **A,** one can see four lesions distinctly (arrows) on the left side (reader's right); the other side of the brain is normal in this slice. In **B,** it is evident that there are numerous lesions on both sides; only the more prominent ones are marked with arrows. The abnormal areas were not visible at all on the CT scan. The lesions are visible on the MRI scan because of a higher water content than surrounding tissue. The patient has minimal disability partly because some of the lesions are in less important regions of the brain and produce no obvious symptoms and partly because functioning nerve fibers still course through the abnormal areas.

In summary, an accurate diagnosis of MS can be made on the basis of characteristic symptoms and confirmatory signs on neurological examination (a detailed examination of the motor system, sensory system, vision, reflexes, etc.). The physician attempts to demonstrate that there are multiple scars (sclerosis) in the CNS for which there is no other explanation, such as strokes or tumors. At times when multiple lesions cannot be demonstrated on neurological examination, or the history of prior attacks cannot be documented, other lesions may be detected by evoked potential testing and MRI. In some cases, spinal fluid examination for oligoclonal bands and immunoglobulins may be necessary for further proof. Only rarely is it necessary to do

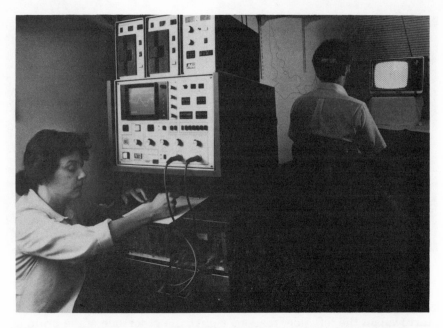

FIG. 1-7. Visual evoked response testing. A technician in the foreground monitors VER testing in a patient who is watching a rapidly reversing checkerboard pattern on a television screen. Electrodes pick up electrical changes in the rear (visual area) of the brain. A computer calculates the average time required for nerve impulses to travel from the retina of the eye to the visual area of the brain. The time is usually prolonged in MS patients.

invasive x-ray procedures such as arteriography or myelography.

Serious errors can be made by relying on symptoms alone or on laboratory tests alone. The diagnosis is usually clinical, with other methods used for confirmation or exclusion of other disorders.

WHO GETS MULTIPLE SCLEROSIS?

MS has occurred in all races, although no cases have yet been reported in the Inuit (Eskimos), and it is rare among the Bantu people.

MS is most common in whites, especially those of northern European ancestry. An *immune response gene* on the sixth human chromosome, called DR2, is common in northern Europeans; it and closely related genes occur in the majority of MS patients, although only a small fraction of persons carrying these genes develop MS. There is some evidence that these genes determine an "overactive" immune system. Antibodies to certain viruses occur in higher titers in DR2+ persons, including patients with MS. Other evidence suggests that common viral infections occur less frequently, and possibly less severely in such persons.

MS occurs more frequently in women than in men; in many clinics the ratio is 2:1. Five percent of MS patients have a brother or sister with MS, and approximately 15% of MS patients have some close relative with the disease.

WHAT IS THE CAUSE OF MULTIPLE SCLEROSIS?

MS is still a disease of unknown cause. Although individuals apparently inherit a tendency to develop the illness, it is not a hereditary disease in the ordinary sense. It is the susceptibility that is inherited. It is rare for a parent and child to be affected in the same family; when one of a pair of identical twins has MS, the other develops manifest illness in less than 50% of cases.

Thus, it seems clear that factors other than heredity are most important. A viral infection has long been under suspicion, but there is little evidence that MS is caused by a virus infecting the nervous system. MS is not contagious: cases in husband and wife are very rare, and have not been seen by most experienced neurologists. Repeated attempts to transmit MS to monkeys and apes have failed, as have attempts to culture a virus in the laboratory; isolated exceptions often receive much publicity, but attempts to duplicate these results have always failed. It is possible to find some viruses in the CNS of people who do not have any evidence of CNS disease.

The most attractive *theory* at the moment is *that MS is an immune ("allergic") reaction in the nervous system.* The provoking agent is uncertain, but detailed studies of large numbers of patients over a period of many years suggest the possibility of an allergic reaction to certain common viruses. Two such studies have now confirmed the fact that *almost one-third of new clinical attacks of MS occur shortly after a cold, influenza, or other common viral illness.* The risk of developing MS with any single virus-like infection is low—about 8–9%, suggesting that all viruses may not have this effect. Which ones do and which do not has not yet been studied adequately. Correlations with changes in the MRI scan in individual patients should hasten progress in this area; it is possible that infection without symptoms (*inapparent infection,* common in partially immune persons) is responsible for many other new lesions.

Some believe that the immune system mistakes for virus a portion of myelin protein that is structurally similar, and destroys it *(molecular mimicry)*. Others have suggested that the viral infection damages myelin and releases small amounts into the circulation, resulting in *autoimmunization.*

One effect of viral infections is to promote the release of *interferon-γ.* Interferon-γ is released by activated T-lymphocytes, and infections promote this activation. Interferon-γ treatment has been shown in one study to increase the frequency of MS attacks dramatically. Immunologists have known for some time that interferon-γ enhances the ability of the immune system to target cells for destruction.

WHAT IS THE NATURAL COURSE OF MULTIPLE SCLEROSIS, WITHOUT TREATMENT?

This, of course, is an important question. It can be answered for groups of patients, but not for an individual patient.

The natural course is highly variable. Sometimes MS produces no symptoms, and is discovered incidentally during an autopsy examination, when the person has died of some other cause. Complete recovery from a first attack is common. Some patients have only two attacks in a lifetime, recover well from each, and never become disabled. Others have rather frequent attacks, and, although not recovering completely each time, still never become totally disabled for productive work (approximately 25% of cases).

Because of this variability, it is impossible to predict with certainty whether a specific person with MS will have mild or severe symptoms in the future.

Many patients eventually have a slow progression of disability, which, over a period of 10–25 years, makes independent walking difficult or impossible. This progression is determined by the intermittent occurrence of new plaques in the brain and spinal cord. Because conduction through new lesions almost always improves, some improvement may be seen from time to time even in this group. Nerve impulses passing through some plaques may be stopped permanently, however, causing symptoms and signs that do not remit (Fig. 1-8).

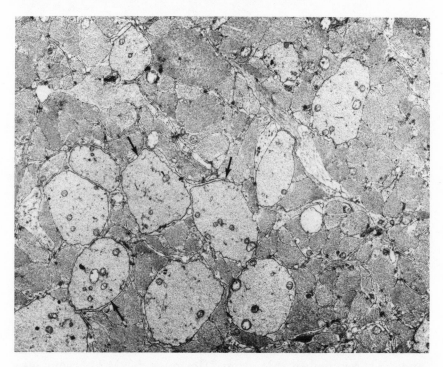

FIG. 1-8. In severe MS, not only is the myelin damaged, but some axons (nerve fibers) are lost also. This electronmicrograph of a plaque shows many demyelinated axons (the large light-colored structures) in the midst of astrocytic scar (the darker structures). Loss of axons, long areas of demyelination, and dense scarring all contribute to making some symptoms permanent.

TABLE 1-1. Progression of Disability in 170 Untreated[a] MS
Patients in One Clinic During a 5-Year Period

DSS at first examination	No. of patients	DSS 5 years later
0	10	0.6
1	22	2.3
2	19	3.4
3	18	4.1
4	14	5.2
5	12	5.8
6	32	6.5
7	28	7.7
8	9	8.3
9	6	9.2

[a]Untreated: during this 5-year observation period, patients received no long-term treatment. Ten to 14 days of adrenocorticotropic hormone or prednisone was often used to treat acute attacks, however.

DSS, Disability Status Scale (the Kurtzke rating): see Table 1-2.

These are average rates of progression: an individual's multiple sclerosis may change less, or more, than the average.

Table 1-1 gives the *average* rate of progression over a period of five years in 170 patients in one clinic. To use the table one must first refer to the *Disability Status Scale (DSS),* to gain some familiarity with the *Kurtzke* DSS scoring system (Table 1-2). Note that DSS scores of 5 or less occur in people who walk independently; those with higher scores require assistance or are in wheelchairs most of the time. Table 1-1 shows that, on average, the natural rate of worsening in MS is slow. For example, among 19 patients who had minimal disability (DSS 2) when first examined, there was a progression to a DSS of 3.4 after 5 years of observation.

A small group of patients have rapid progression to major disability over a period of months or a few years. Life expectancy is shortened in this group. However, for MS persons as a whole, life expectancy is near normal. There is no accurate method of predicting the course of any individual person with MS. However, if a long time passes since diagnosis without significant disability, this usually means a milder future course for the illness.

TABLE 1-2. Disability Status Scale (DSS—Kurtzke) (Highly simplified and abbreviated)

Rating	Status
0	Normal neurological examination
1	No disability, minimal abnormal signs on examination
2	Minimal disability in only one of the following functional systems: strength, coordination, sensation, bladder, vision, mental
3	Walking independently, but moderate disability in one of the functional systems (above)
4	Walking independently, up 12 h a day, but severe disability in one functional system
5	Walking without aid for 200 m, but disability severe enough to prevent working a full day
6	Cane, crutch, or brace required to walk 100 m
7	Walking limited to 5 m with aid; mostly confined to wheelchair
8	Confined to bed or chair; effective use of arms
9	Helpless bed patient
10	Death from MS

HOW IS THE PROGRESS OF MULTIPLE SCLEROSIS MEASURED?

Accurate methods of measurement are essential in all research. Methods for quantitating the progress of MS in an individual patient, or in a group of patients, therefore assume importance. A number of scoring systems have been devised. We have already referred to the DSS rating system, the one used most commonly by neurologists to quantitate degree of disability. Another scoring system called *Minimal Record of Disability (MRD)* was developed by the International Federation of Multiple Sclerosis Societies (IFMSS) and is now being widely used to supplement the DSS system; among other things, it scores handicaps in activities of daily living, and socioeconomic disability. Several portions of the MRD do not require a neurological examination and can be administered by nurses, psychologists, physiotherapists, and other nonphysician health professionals.

Recently, more accurate assessment of activity and extent of MS in an individual patient has been made possible by the MRI scan. To the present time MRI has been used primarily to aid in diagnosis, but it is also ideally suited to follow the progress of the illness, and monitor the effect of treatment—because it can detect new plaques that do not produce new symptoms or any changes on examination. A treatment that prevents the appearance of new lesions on MRI in a substantial number of patients over a period of time would quickly be established as effective. So far, none of the recommended therapies has been shown to have this ability.

II

History, Rationale, and Summary of Treatments in Multiple Sclerosis

More research to find the cause of MS is being done now than at any other time in history. Perhaps when the exact cause is found it will lead quickly to a cure. Now, however, as in the past, most treatments for MS are based on the latest ideas about causation. In the 1930s for example, some thought MS was caused by infection by a spirochete; fever therapy was then used in some cases, because another neurological illness caused by a spirochete was benefited by this treatment. MS was not helped by fever treatment, and few now believe that it is caused by a spirochete.

This chapter discusses the special problems in evaluating treatment in MS, and some of the old and current theories about its cause, as well as briefly summarizing results with each major type of treatment (see also page 11: What Is the Cause of Multiple Sclerosis?).

PROBLEMS IN EVALUATION OF THERAPY

The variability of multiple sclerosis in different people, and its tendency to improve without treatment, has made evaluation of therapy especially difficult. Before 1960, at least 43 reports described "successes" in treatment that are now known to be nothing more than descriptions of the natural course of the illness. The ability of MS to show dramatic improvement without therapy has deceived many well-meaning physicians and laymen into believing they had discovered a "cure."

Table 2-1 outlines the results of treatment with 15 different types of treatment used from 1935–1950. The majority of the 435 patients improved (66%). Nevertheless, these same methods of treatment are seldom, if ever, used now because further experience has shown them to be no better than no therapy. Other careful studies have shown that when patients are treated for recent worsening, 70% improve on placebo medication. Stated more simply, *the use of a completely ineffective treatment in patients with recent worsening is associated with improvement in 65–70% of patients.* Thus, any new treatment for recent progression of MS must produce sustained improvement in more than 70% of patients to attract the attention of experienced physicians.

When prophylactic treatment has been used over a period of several years in uncontrolled studies, ineffective agents often register the following results: one-third improved, one-third the same, and one-third worse.

TABLE 2-1. Summary of Treatments from 1935–1950, by Rationale or Mode of Application

Rationale or application	No. of agents	No. of patients	No. improved	% Improved
Antiallergic	2	169	126	75%
Anticoagulant	1	43	30	70
Physical	3	15	12	80
Vasodilator	4	140	87	62
Vitamins	5	68	30	44
Totals	15	435	285	66%

Range of frequency of improvement with individual agents	0–100%
Range of improvement other than 0 and 100%	31–90%

Another way of judging treatment efficacy in MS is to ask: Can this method prevent worsening? A *completely effective treatment* would stop worsening in all cases, and probably produce improvement in most patients, and would be easy to recognize. A controlled trial of therapy would not be necessary. Unfortunately, no such agent has been discovered.

PROPER TREATMENT TRIALS

The recognition of a *partially effective treatment* requires the use of control patients treated simultaneously with placebo. In a *controlled trial of therapy*, treated and control patients should be entered randomly into the trial so that the average condition of patients in the two groups is similar. In a well-randomized trial, for example, there will be the same number of patients with red hair, and weakness of the left leg, and the average duration of the illness in the two groups will be similar. Randomization avoids the tendency that an enthusiastic therapist might otherwise have of unconsciously assigning more severely ill patients to the control group, thus biasing the study in favor of the treated group.

A properly controlled trial should ideally also be *blinded*. In a *single-blind* trial the patient is not told whether placebo or active drug is being administered; this ensures that the same enthusiasm and hope will be present in both groups, factors known to improve performance in anyone.

A preferred design is to have neither the patient nor the physician who evaluates the patient's progress know which treatment is given *(double-blind study);* this avoids reporting bias due to overenthusiasm on the part of the treating physician. In double-blind trials one physician, who does not participate in evaluation of drug efficacy, is aware of the treatment being given, and closely watches patient safety during the trial.

Controlled trials of treatment speed up the search for an effective treatment. They are difficult to organize because more than one clinic usually must be involved *(a multicenter trial)* to ensure adequate numbers of patients. The detailed care required and extensive record keeping are also expensive. Nonetheless, it has been shown that therapies can be evaluated in reasonable periods of time—often 2–3 years—using such trials. Many years ago, before such trials were used, useless treatments often continued to be used for as long as 15 years: examples are the anticoagulant, dicumarol, and the blood vessel dilator, histamine. Since about 1960 most treatment trials have been controlled, and medical journals usually refuse to publish the results of uncontrolled treatment.

Some recent trials of treatment not only are controlled, but also use the MRI scan, repeated frequently in patients and controls. Many new lesions seen on MRI are unassociated with new symptoms, and in the past would have gone undetected. Treatments incapable of preventing new lesions detected with MRI can be discarded quickly, and more promising treatments tried. Proper use of the MRI scan should thus speed up the search for curative treatment. MRI scanners dedicated to MS research and paid for by MS research funds are needed to accelerate the pace of research.

RATIONALE AND SUMMARY OF TREATMENTS, OLD AND RECENT

The historical rationale for trying the many and various treatments for MS can be summarized under the headings of: (a) that it is a *metabolic abnormality;* (b) that MS is due to a *circulatory insufficiency;* (c) that it is due to *improper diet;* (d) that it is an *infection;* (e) that *anti-inflammatory drugs might help* because inflammation is seen in early plaques; (f) that it is a *disorder of the immune system.* A final rationale is *an empiric one:* (g) that the cause remains unknown but trial and error indicates that certain methods may be effective. Many old treatments are no longer used (Table 2-2).

Metabolic Abnormalities

The concept that metabolic abnormalities might account for the development of MS can be traced back at least to 1916. This is currently regarded as unlikely, because the lesions of MS are

TABLE 2-2. Some MS Treatments Chiefly of Historical Interest[a]

Theory of metabolic disturbance
  Adenosine 5'-monophosphate
  Cocarboxylase
  Cytochrome C
  Digestive enzymes
  Galactose
  Sodium succinate
  Tolbutamide

Theory of circulatory disturbance
  Atromid-S
  Dicumarol
  Heparin[b]
  Histamine
  Hydergine
  Tetraethylammonium chloride

Infection theory
  Adenine arabinoside
  Autogenous vaccines
  Cytosine arabinoside
  Gamma globulins
  Hyperimmune colostrum
  Nystatin
  Russian vaccine
  Staphlococcal vaccines
  Whole blood transfusions

Theory of immune disturbance
  Fever therapy
  Foreign protein
  Typhoid vaccine
  Piromen
  Intrathecal tuberculin
  Thoracic duct drainage
  Thymectomy
  Transfer factor

[a]Some of the methods included in this table continue to be reviewed in more detail elsewhere in this volume because of their general interest or recent use. Readers interested in more information about some of the other methods should consult the index, the previous edition, or selected references on page 189.

[b]Heparin is still under investigation because of certain effects of the drug on the immune system, but not because of its anticoagulant properties.

discrete, scattered, asymmetric, and inflammatory. Known metabolic disorders affecting the nervous system, by contrast, are usually associated with diffuse symmetric, noninflammatory degeneration of nerve cells or nerve fibers. Furthermore, *no metabolic or biochemical changes have been found consistently in MS.*

The major theories in the past suggested a defect in carbohydrate metabolism; alterations, such as decreased glucose tolerance, were reported in some patients; in retrospect, however, these changes correlated best with physical inactivity or poor nutrition, rather than with MS itself. Agents used in a more-or-less blind attempt to correct hypothetical defects in metabolism include sodium succinate, cocarboxylase, tolbutamide, galactose, adenosine 5'-monophosphate (My-B-Den), cytochrome C, and digestive enzymes. *These agents are seldom, if ever, used today.*

Circulatory Insufficiency

Another hypothesis current 30–40 years ago was that MS was caused by poor circulation in parts of the CNS. One idea proposed that clots forming in small veins caused the illness; another proposed that sluggish blood flow had the same effect. A number of therapies were used for many years based on these theories, which now have few believers: anticoagulant drugs (dicumarol, heparin), the low-fat diet, blood vessel dilating drugs (vasodilators) such as histamine, tetraethylammonium (TEA) chloride, Hydergine, papaverine, amyl nitrite, aminophylline, belladonna, alcohol, diphenhydramine (Benadryl), tripelennamine (Pyribenzamine), benzazoline (Priscoline), and nicotinic acid (niacin). More recent additions to drugs of this class include the calcium-channel-blocking drugs: verapamil, nifedipine, and diltiazem.

In the opinion of the Therapeutic Claims Committee, *there is no convincing evidence of favorable effect due to anticoagulants or vasodilators, alone or in combination, on the natural course of MS.* The same can be said of circulatory stimulants such as caffeine and ephedrine, and physical means of stimulating circulation in the skin and muscles, such as by the alternate use of cold and pressure, and heat and massage.

Diet

There is no established nutritional deficiency in MS patients. Persons with MS need a well-balanced diet as much as others, but no convincing evidence exists that the addition of vitamins, even in high doses, or minerals alters the course of MS.

Because the geographical areas of prevalence of MS are also high-fat-consuming areas of the world, some have proposed a low-fat diet. In the past, high-fat diets have been used "to protect the myelin," which is a fatty substance. Others have proposed gluten-free diets, raw-food diets, and supplementation with polyunsaturated fatty acids (PUFA): linolenic acid, linoleic acid, sunflower seed oil, safflower seed oil, evening primrose oil (Naudicelle, Gamma Prim), and fish oil.

PUFA have some slight immunosuppressive properties. Sunflower seed oil, evening primrose oil, and safflower seed oil have been tested. One controlled study reported some reduction in frequency of exacerbations. Another reported some reduction in the severity and duration of attacks, but no change in their frequency; a third study found no effect. A large controlled trial of fish oil in Great Britain, recently completed, showed a trend in favor of the fish-oil-treated patients. Other than a possible benefit of PUFA-containing oils, there is no evidence that any other dietary change affects MS.

Although the preponderance of evidence suggests that the effect of diet in MS is very limited, if present at all, this edition continues to describe many of the diets that have been recommended, because of continued strong patient interest in this topic.

Infection

As noted in the Introduction (see page 11: What Is the Cause of Multiple Sclerosis?), there is little to support the idea that the areas of damage in MS are the direct result of viral infection, or the direct effects of any other infectious agent. However, there are at least two recent prospective studies suggesting that viral infections are a major risk factor and can trigger exacerbations.

Interferon-α and interferon-β have both been reported to reduce the frequency of exacerbations. If this is true, the mechanism is not clear; these interferons could, however, reduce the frequency of common viral infections suspected of triggering attacks. Other antiviral drugs have been used, e.g., acyclovir, amantadine, and Isoprinosine, but there is still inadequate data to judge their effects.

Interferon-γ, as noted in the Introduction, apparently worsens MS and, in the opinion of the Committee, should not be used; interferon-inducing drugs should also be avoided because many of them induce the production of interferon-γ.

Vaccines have been made from viruses allegedly grown from some MS brains, e.g., the Russian vaccine; the treatment is not effective in MS. A number of other methods have been based on unproven hypotheses that MS is caused by various molds, rickettsiae, or other agents. These include nystatin, autogenous vaccines, staphylococcal vaccines, and Le Gac therapy (anti-rickettsial treatment with tetracycline antibiotics) and are now chiefly of historical interest. Certain antiviral drugs intended to treat herpesvirus infections, such as adenine arabinoside (Ara-A) and cytosine arabinoside (Ara-C) were apparently never systematically tried in MS, and have been eliminated from the present edition because a safer and more effective anti-herpesvirus drug (acyclovir) now exists.

Inflammation

Most tissues recover well after an inflammatory response, for example, from infection or allergic reaction. CNS tissue, however, contains elements (nerve cells, myelin) that regenerate poorly if at all. The acute MS plaque is inflammatory and swollen, with dilated, leaky blood vessels, and the tissues are infiltrated with inflammatory cells from the blood (lymphocytes, macrophages), some of which participate in causing the damage, some of which help limit the damage and clean up after it.

The improvements seen in MS are frequent and often dramatic. Much of the improvement is thought to be due to a subsidence of swelling and inflammation. Drugs that promote this antiinflammatory response are adrenocorticotropic hormone (ACTH), prednisone, methlyprednisolone, and beta- and dexamethasone. Such agents have been shown to shorten the duration of an acute MS bout in a modest way. In doses that can be tolerated for long periods, they have not been shown to prevent new attacks or alter the course of MS.

Immune System

The concept that persons with MS may have an overactive or unusual immune system has already been discussed (see page 11 in the Introduction). Advances in the understanding of the immune system continue to occur at a rapid rate and will undoubtedly lead to the trial of new treatments.

Currently the most commonly used methods intended to slow the rate of worsening of MS are the immunosuppressive drugs (azathioprine, cyclophosphamide, cyclosporine). Total lymphoid irradiation has shown promising results in one study. Other studies have attempted to desensitize patients to a hypothetical allergen, myelin basic protein (MBP), by injecting a non–illness-producing synthetic analog resembling a portion of the MBP molecule (copolymer I). Other procedures used in an attempt to alter the immune response are plasmapheresis and lymphocytapheresis. Prednisone and similar drugs are also immunosuppressive.

The complete results of a large cooperative study of cyclosporine and azathioprine should be announced later in 1988. Azathioprine has been disappointing in short-term use (1–2 years), but many physicians experienced in its use believe it dampens the severity of MS after longer use. The evidence about the effectiveness of cyclophosphamide is conflicting; earlier reports suggested it had the ability to stabilize steadily progressive illness for 1–2 years, but other studies found no difference in treated and control subjects, especially if proper blinding was maintained during the trial.

A small controlled study of copolymer I (COP-I) showed an

apparent benefit in reducing attacks in the remitting–exacerbating form of the illness, but most, including ourselves, believe that further confirmatory tests are necessary. Unfortunately COP-I is not available, and until it becomes available additional studies cannot be done.

The use of plasmapheresis, usually in combination with immunosuppressive drugs, has been reported to have a beneficial effect in small controlled studies. There still is no consensus, however, that this very expensive procedure is effective.

Empirical Treatments: No Good Scientific Rationale

Although medical science always tries to be scientific and totally rational, it has a rich history of success born of dogged persistence and the empiric (trial and error) approach. This approach continues in MS, with the hope that better educated guesses about agents to try are likely now, due to progress in many other scientific areas, especially immunology.

Methods in this category are a miscellaneous assortment of treatments that either have no scientific rationale, based on our present knowledge, or a weak rationale. Many old treatments for MS were based on the fact that a few patients using a medication (or diet) for some other reason showed improvement in MS symptoms. Examples include the following: the MacDougal diet, tolbutamide, isoniazid. None of these methods are now considered effective.

Useful medicines have been discovered by trial and error in the past, and inclusion in this category does not necessarily mean that the methods deserve no consideration.

CONTINUING PROBLEMS IN TREATMENT TRIALS

As emphasized earlier, the preferred method for evaluating the usefulness of treatments in MS is the controlled trial. How can one explain, then, the occasional announcement of positive results in a trial that others later cannot duplicate?

An example is treatment with hyperbaric oxygen. One trial reported good results, but several studies subsequently could not show benefit. One possible reason is that the numbers of patients were inadequate in the earlier study. Improper blinding is sometimes a cause of conflicting results: a well-meaning but enthusiastic physician may develop an emotional attachment to a therapy; if the doctor or patient knows through subtle clues, in spite of precautions, that the patient is not receiving placebo, a more favorable rating may be given.

Another example is the conflicting reports concerning cyclophosphamide. This drug was originally reported to be capable of stabilizing progressive MS for periods of up to 2 years. Blinding was impossible during the earlier studies, because all patients temporarily became bald as a side effect of the treatment. A later controlled study was blinded by having the evaluating physician examine the patient before treatment, and again only after hair had regrown. In this latest study no benefit from the drug could be found.

Evaluation of cyclophosphamide in controlled studies continues, in the hope that the true place of this agent may be discovered by the use of larger numbers of patients.

A POLL OF THE COMMITTEE

In mid-1987, the members of the Therapeutic Claims Committee were asked the following questions:

1. *Major acute exacerbation of MS:* My preference for treatment includes:

        ☐   Bed rest
        ☐   ACTH gel
        ☐   Prednisone
        ☐   Dexamethasone or betamethasone
        ☐   Other

The results were as follows:

ACTH or i.v. methylprednisolone	1
Prednisone	3

Prednisone, dexamethasone,
   or betamethasone   1
Dexamethasone or betametha-
   sone   4
i.v. methylprednisolone   <u>1</u>
                                      10

2. *A patient slowly progressive from the onset of disease, who
   has never shown natural improvement, worsening by at least
   one DSS point per year.* My preferred treatment would be:

   □   Intermittent ACTH gel
   □   Alternate day prednisone
   □   Azathioprine
   □   Azathioprine + prednisone
   □   Cyclosporine
   □   Cyclophosphamide
   □   Plasma exchange with or without
         immunosuppressive drugs
   □   No drug treatment
   □   Copolymer I
   □   Other; please specify.

The responses were as follows:

Intermittent ACTH gel   0
Alternate day prednisone   1
Azathioprine + prednisone   3 (one
                                      specified low-dose
                                      prednisone)

Azathioprine or
   cyclophosphamide   1
Plasma exchange   0
Cyclosporine   0
i.v. methylprednisolone for 1–8
   days   1
i.v. methylprednisolone followed
   by azathioprine   1

High dose prednisone,
　　a clinical trial if it fails　　　　　　2
No drug treatment, refer to a
　　clinical trial　　　　　　　　　　1
Copolymer I　　　　　　　　　　　 0
　　　　　　　　　　　　　　　　 ——
　　　　　　　　　　　　　　　　 10

The editor who would use azathioprine *or* cyclophophamide would not use them together, or sequentially, and would use antilymphocytic globulin in a severe case if cyclophosphamide was refused. Another editor would try cyclophosphamide, as a second choice after azathioprine or azathioprine + prednisone, if these failed.

The results show that all of these neurologists with wide experience in MS use corticosteroids during major new attacks; they also show that for relentlessly progressive disease, prednisone or methylprednisolone is used, at least for brief periods; azathioprine is used by half of the editors in their own practices, with two using cyclophosphamide in very severe cases.

III

Treatment for an Acute Exacerbation

OVERVIEW

At least 80–85% of MS patients at some time have an acute period of worsening (also called exacerbation, bout, attack, or relapse). MRI scans taken at such times may show new lesions in the CNS or enlargement of old ones. The variety of symptoms possible in such acute exacerbations has already been discussed (see page 5 in the Introduction).

Improvement usually occurs naturally after an acute bout, most commonly in 4–12 weeks. The degree of natural improvement varies as described on page 12 of the Introduction. The reasons for improvement are not completely understood, but much of it is undoubtedly due to a reduction in inflammation.

The principal drugs used to treat acute exacerbations are those having major antiinflammatory properties: ACTH and synthetic adrenal steroids, such as prednisone, methylprednisolone, betamethasone, and dexamethasone.

ACTH has been shown in studies from 20 years ago to shorten the duration of exacerbations by an estimated 10–15%. The pharmacological effects of the other drugs mentioned are similar to those of ACTH, although they are more potent, cause less sodium retention, less potassium loss, and have a longer duration of action. Recently claims have been made that intravenous methylprednisolone in high doses works faster than ACTH, and many physicians now prefer this drug in treatment of acute attacks.

All the above-mentioned drugs have possible serious side-effects, and should only be used under the supervision of a physician. Although these agents are widely used in acute attacks of MS, there is no good evidence that they alter the extent of residual disability, and their use is contraindicated in patients in whom they produce psychosis or other serious side-effects.

Other antiinflammatory drugs, the so-called nonsteroidal antiinflammatory drugs (NSAIDs), include aspirin, indomethacin, ibuprofen, naproxen, and others. These drugs have not been shown to be of benefit in MS, and one, indomethacin, has been reported to make it worse. Because of this, most of these NSAIDs should probably be avoided by MS patients, unless their physicians determine otherwise. Aspirin would appear to be safe, but further studies are necessary to clarify the action of the other NSAIDs in MS.

INFLAMMATION: ADRENOCORTICOTROPIC HORMONE AND ADRENAL CORTICOSTEROIDS

Adrenocorticotropic Hormone, Synthetic Adrenal Glucocorticoids (Prednisone, Prednisolone, Methylprednisolone, Betamethasone, Dexamethasone)

Description: ACTH is a protein hormone extracted from the pituitary glands of animals; synthetic analogs are also available. It must be given by injection, and acts by stimulating the adrenal gland to release glucocorticoid hormones, most of which are now made synthetically. The synthetic glucocorticoids are more potent, cause less sodium retention, less potassium loss, and have a longer duration of action than ACTH.

Rationale: These agents reduce edema and other aspects of inflammation, chiefly by inhibiting a phospholipase enzyme that is the first step in the production of inflammation after tissue injury. They also have an effect on T-lymphocytes and have some immunosuppressive properties. The drugs also cause a temporary improvement in nerve conduction through demyelinated areas, and often produce a mild euphoria and a sense of increased energy.

Evaluation: Short-term ACTH given daily in high doses has been reported to reduce the severity of individual MS attacks. A short-term (1-month) study was completed 20 years ago that was a well randomized, double-blind trial in several clinical centers. The positive result obtained is widely accepted; the effect was to shorten the duration of an acute exacerbation modestly, about 10–15%. In more recent smaller controlled studies, claims have been made that high-dose intravenous methylprednisolone works more quickly and effectively than ACTH. The drug is usually given as a 5-day course, and its use is now common practice in many clinics and hospitals.

The long-term use of ACTH or synthetic adrenal hormones has shown that, when given in modest daily doses that can be tolerated for long periods, they do not alter the frequency of exacerbations or limit progression. Given in high doses for long periods they cause a high rate of complications, and this factor limits such treatment. Side-effects can be minimized to some extent by using prednisone on alternate days, in moderate or high doses for months or even years. *Betamethasone and dexamethasone are not suitable for alternate-day use because of long half-lives.* One small controlled study of alternate-day therapy with prednisone found a reduced number of exacerbations compared with placebo-treated patients. This type of treatment is often used in severe MS, especially in patients who relapse shortly after discontinuing short-term treatment.

Risks/Costs: The complications of short- and long-term treatment with these agents are well established. Complications include: generalized puffiness, "moon face," psychosis, peptic ulceration, infections, and acne. With long-term use, fractures due to bone softening, aseptic necrosis of bone, cataracts, hypertension, and adrenal insufficiency may occur. There have also been observations suggesting that neurologic worsening may occur shortly after therapy is stopped or reduced below a certain level.

Patients receiving intravenous methylprednisolone must be under close medical supervision, because rare but serious reactions have been reported. Some patients with heart disease should not use this form of treatment.

In addition to the cost of medication, one must consider the cost of repeated laboratory tests for possible complications.

Conclusion: Short-term high-dose therapy with these drugs is effective in many patients in shortening exacerbations of MS and reducing their severity. Long-term, daily, moderate-dose treatment does not change the natural course of MS, whereas long-term high dose therapy carries a high risk of complications. Long-term alternate-day therapy reduces the risk of complications, but effectiveness has not been documented.

In the opinion of the Committee, the efficacy of this therapy in selected patients has been demonstrated. Long-term use may be associated with significant serious side-effects.

INFLAMMATION: ADRENOCORTICOTROPHIC HORMONE AND ADRENAL CORTICOSTEROIDS

Intrathecal Synthetic Corticosteroids

Description: This treatment involves the injection of *methylprednisolone* (Depo-Medrol) or similar agents by lumbar puncture into the cerebrospinal fluid (CSF).

Rationale: It was thought that this procedure brings the injected drug to the MS lesions directly and at higher concentrations than administration by other routes, although this has never been proved.

Evaluation: Intrathecal steroids have been used as a treatment for MS for approximately 20 years. Originally, there were claims of improvement in spasticity, gait, and sphincter control, and even of complete remissions. Several later reports, however, have failed to show improvement. Indeed, it has not been established that intrathecal injection actually does result in higher levels of drug at the sites of disease.

Risks/Costs: Infections of the meninges, as well as arachnoiditis (inflammation and adhesions of the subarachnoid space, in which the CSF circulates) have been reported.

Conclusion: Most neurologists no longer use, or never have used, intrathecal steroids because of the hazards and the lack of convincing evidence of increased effectiveness.

In the opinion of the Committee, this therapy should not be used because of reported harmful effects.

INFLAMMATION: AGENTS AFFECTING PROSTAGLANDIN PATHWAYS

Aspirin and Sodium Salicylate

Description: Aspirin is well known as a pain reliever and is available without a prescription.

Rationale: Both aspirin and sodium salicylate have moderate antiinflammatory effects, and have been employed in rheumatoid arthritis. Their main effect is to inhibit enzymes involved in the synthesis of prostaglandins. The latter are lipid hormones that are released during inflammation, some of which increase the inflammatory response. Prostaglandin E_2, however, has antiinflammatory properties.

Evaluation: Sodium salicylate was first reported as a treatment for MS in 1926. There are two reports of its use in MS. In a controlled trial with heavy doses of soluble aspirin over a 14-month period, the treated group did no better or worse than did controls.

Risks/Costs: These agents are inexpensive but tend to produce peptic ulceration and gastrointestinal bleeding as a side effect; this effect is more marked if they are given to patients who are also receiving ACTH or synthetic adrenal corticosteroids, a practice best avoided.

Conclusion: Aspirin does not appear to help or worsen MS. It may be used for pain. *Acetaminophen* may be preferred for this purpose, because it is not a prostaglandin inhibitor and does not cause stomach irritation.

In the opinion of the Committee, this therapy has been adequately tested and shown to be without value. It is relatively free of serious adverse side-effects during short-term use.

INFLAMMATION: AGENTS AFFECTING PROSTAGLANDIN PATHWAYS

Nonsteroidal Antiinflammatory Drugs: Indomethacin (Indocin), phenylbutazone (Butazolidin), naproxen (Naprosyn), sulindac (Clinoril), ibuprofen (Advil, Motrin), fenoprofen (Nalfon), tolmetin (Tolectin), ketoprofen (Orudis), and others

Description: NSAIDs are synthetic chemicals that inhibit prostaglandin synthesis. Some inhibit certain prostaglandins more than others. Some prostaglandins contribute to inflammation; some, such as prostaglandin E, however, may inhibit inflammation, and have immunosuppressive properties as well.

Rationale: These substances are widely used in medicine to reduce inflammation, especially in arthritis. Some are effective to varying degrees in the animal model of experimental allergic encephalomyelitis (EAE) (see page 50: The Immune System and Multiple Sclerosis) but indomethacin has been reported to make EAE worse.

Evaluation: Proper evaluation of this class of drugs in MS has not been done. One study, however, suggests that indomethacin makes MS worse. There are theoretical reasons why this might happen, but it is impossible to predict what the result of each of the many drugs in this series might have on MS, based on what is known of their chemistry.

Conclusion: Because of uncertainties about the effects of these drugs on MS, caution in their use is suggested until the situation is clarified.

In the opinion of the Committee, there appears to be no generally accepted scientific basis for use of this therapy. It has never been tested in a proper controlled trial.

INFLAMMATION: PROTEASE INHIBITORS

Epsilon Aminocaproic Acid

Description: Epsilon aminocaproic acid (EACA) is a simple chemical molecule that inhibits the activity of certain enzymes that digest protein.

Rationale: The developing plaque of MS contains large numbers of macrophages (scavenger cells), which appear to destroy myelin by digesting its proteins and lipids. Inhibitors of the enzymes responsible for this digestion might reduce the myelin destruction or even interfere with movement of the macrophages into and through the tissues. EACA suppresses lesions in the animal model EAE very effectively. Because this drug has been safely used in other conditions (transplantation of normal tissues, surgery on tumors), it seems appropriate to consider clinical trials in MS. Other naturally derived or synthetic compounds such as pepstatin with similar activity have been shown to inhibit EAE, but have not yet been considered for use in MS. Still others *(leupeptin, antipain, chymostatin, bestatin, amastatin, esterastin)* are being tested in Japan in various inflammatory disorders and are also of potential interest for use in MS.

Evaluation: A small number of patients have been treated with EACA in a pilot study. Those with relapsing disease of recent onset and with mild disease appeared to show rapid improvement. The treatment also appeared to be effective in patients with acute encephalitis from other causes. There have been no follow-up studies in the last four years.

Risk/Costs: EACA has been used in subarachnoid hemorrhage, and complications observed included thrombotic state, delirium, weakness, and myopathy. Relatively low doses were used for encephalitis and in MS patients, and no complications were observed.

Conclusion: Insufficient evidence exists on which to base a recommendation.

In the opinion of the Committee, the rationale of this therapy is plausible, but the results of controlled trials are not yet available, and it must be regarded as investigational.

INFLAMMATION: MISCELLANEOUS ANTIINFLAMMATORY AGENTS

Desferrioxamine Mesylate (Desferal)

Description: This is a simple drug that serves as a highly specific chelating (binding) agent for iron. It is widely used, by repeated intramuscular or subcutaneous injection, in iron-overload diseases such as thalassemia and hemochromatosis.

Rationale: A major cause of tissue damage in inflammatory lesions such as those found in MS may be free oxygen, hydroxyl radicals, superoxide, and hydrogen peroxide, which are produced by the activated macrophages in the lesions. Formation of these requires the presence of metals such as iron and can be inhibited by chelating agents such as desferrioxamine. Desferrioxamine also inhibits lymphocytic reactions.

Evaluation: In rats, desferrioxamine inhibits autoimmune encephalomyelitis and accelerates recovery when treatment is started after disease is already present. The drug is now being tested in MS in pilot studies in Australia and larger trials are planned in Australia and the United States.

Risks/Costs: The need to give desferrioxamine by injection and the short duration of its effect are serious drawbacks. However, oral, long-lasting, iron-chelating drugs similar to desferrioxamine are being developed. High doses have been associated with ocular and auditory abnormalities.

Conclusion: Desferrioxamine is a potentially interesting, relatively nontoxic agent for trial in MS. The results of current trials are awaited with interest.

In the opinion of the Committee, the rationale of this therapy is plausible, but it has not been adequately tested, and must be regarded as experimental. Long-term use may be associated with significant serious side-effects.

INFLAMMATION: MISCELLANEOUS ANTIINFLAMMATORY AGENTS

Chloroquine

Description: Chloroquine is an antimalarial agent that is available by prescription.

Rationale: Chloroquine has been used in the treatment of rheumatoid arthritis and related inflammatory disorders.

Evaluation: A controlled study over a period of 14 months showed no benefit from the use of chloroquine in MS.

Risks/Costs: The most threatening aspect of chloroquine use is permanent visual loss from retinal degeneration. This may begin to develop as early as 3 to 6 months after beginning treatment.

Conclusion: The absence of demonstrated benefit from chloroquine in MS and the risk of visual loss appear to contraindicate its use as a treatment.

In the opinion of the Committee, this therapy should not be used because of reported harmful effects. Long-term use may be associated with significant serious side-effects.

INFLAMMATION: MISCELLANEOUS ANTIINFLAMMATORY AGENTS

D-Penicillamine

Description: This is a simple compound extracted from certain fungi.

Rationale: D-Penicillamine is a compound that has been used in some autoimmune diseases, such as rheumatoid arthritis. Penicillamine was also shown experimentally to be active against certain neurotropic viruses. Both activities justify trials of agents of this type for MS.

Evaluation: There have been two uncontrolled trials of penicillamine in Poland and one in the United States. In one, exacerbations were not decreased and progression was not prevented. Two of the trials reported improvement in some patients.

Risks/Costs: Toxic effects observed included: general weakness, skin rash, decreased blood platelets, kidney damage, and disturbance of electrolyte balance (low potassium).

Conclusion: D-Penicillamine has not been assessed by properly designed clinical trials; however, the reported failure of D-penicillamine to prevent exacerbation and progression suggests that this drug is not a promising treatment.

In the opinion of the Committee, the rationale of this therapy is plausible, but it has not been adequately tested, and must be regarded as experimental. Long-term use may be associated with significant serious side-effects.

INFLAMMATION: MISCELLANEOUS ANTIINFLAMMATORY AGENTS

Nervous System Irradiation (X-ray)

Description: Irradiation of the central nervous system.

Rationale: This procedure was used for its antiinflammatory effect or, possibly, as an "antiinfective" measure.

Evaluation: Irradiation of the CNS was first reported in 1903, and by 1932, 316 MS patients had been so treated. Improvement was seen in 45%, a rate comparable to that seen with numerous ineffective therapies. Additional reports continued as late as 1970 (see page 62: Total Lymphoid Irradiation).

Risks/Costs: Comparable to those of x-ray therapy for other diseases, such as tumors.

Conclusion: On the basis of the published evidence, this treatment should be considered ineffective in MS.

In the opinion of the Committee, this therapy has been adequately tested and shown to be without value. Its use carries significant risk.

INFLAMMATION: MISCELLANEOUS
ANTIINFLAMMATORY AGENTS

Mannitol

Description: Mannitol is a simple sugar, which, when given in a high dose intravenously, can be effective temporarily in reducing edema (fluid which has leaked into the brain) in the presence of a damaged blood–brain barrier.

Rationale: CT and MRI scanning have demonstrated fluid leakage from damaged vessels in the acute brain lesions of MS. Agents that slow or reverse the movement of fluid should reduce the associated neurologic abnormalities.

Evaluation: Careful double-blind controlled studies have shown significant reduction in acute MS symptomatology in patients given a large dose of intravenous mannitol. However, benefit was short-lived (minutes to hours) and led to no apparent long-term advantage.

Risks/Costs: "Rebound" effects are not uncommon in other forms of cerebral edema after short-term use of mannitol.

Conclusion: Mannitol produces transient improvement in acute MS but is not considered by the Committee to offer a useful form of therapy.

In the opinion of the Committee, the rationale of this therapy is plausible, but the results of controlled trials are not yet available, and it must be regarded as investigational. It is relatively free of serious adverse side-effects during short-term use.

INFLAMMATION: AGENTS AFFECTING CATECHOLAMINE PATHWAYS

Prazosin and Similar Agents

Description: Prazosin is one of a group of drugs that mimic and/ or antagonize the actions of catecholamines, the physiologic mediators that regulate blood flow. Technically it is known as an α-adrenergic receptor antagonist. It is used as an antihypertensive agent.

Rationale: Because the lesions of MS and those of the animal model disease EAE begin with inflammation in and around blood vessels, it is of interest to test agents that act on vessels for their possible effect on lesion development. Prazosin may act either as a vasodilator or, in some situations, a vasoconstrictor. It is also thought to act on lymphocyte function (not well studied). In any case, it strongly suppresses EAE. By contrast, two other vasoconstrictive agents, *yohimbine,* an α_2-adrenergic blocker, and *propranolol,* a β-adrenergic blocker, both acted to increase the intensity of EAE.

Evaluation: A trial of prazosin is the planning stage.

Risks/Costs: The drug is inexpensive and has few side-effects other than dizziness, lethargy, and a sudden fall of blood pressure when it is first administered.

Conclusion: The results of planned trials are awaited with interest.

In the opinion of the Committee, the rationale of this therapy is plausible, but it has not been adequately tested, and must be regarded as experimental. It is relatively free of serious adverse side-effects during long-term use.

IV

Methods Used to Prevent Worsening of Multiple Sclerosis

OVERVIEW

Immunosuppressive drugs are those that dampen most or certain aspects of the immune system. Some, such as azathioprine and cyclophosphamide, either kill or prevent the formation of lymphocytes. Cyclosporine seems to have a selective effect in inhibiting T-helper lymphocytes. The use of these drugs is associated with potentially serious side-effects, and they are not suitable for use in mild or very slowly progressive MS. Current evidence suggests that azathioprine in long-term use may dampen the severity of MS in a modest way, but it produces little immediate benefit. Cyclophosphamide has greater toxicity, and although some believe it can slow the progress of MS, other studies have been unable to confirm this; its use should probably be restricted to rapidly progressive cases not responding to other methods, and then preferably in the setting of a clinical trial. The results of several cyclosporine trials are still not completely known: however, initial indications are that both the United Kingdom–Dutch and U.S. trials seem to show a benefit in comparison with placebo, but the extent of the benefits and whether they outweigh risks await further data analysis; the German cyclosporine trial was able to find no advantage of cyclosporine over azathioprine.

Immune modulators are substances capable of altering the function of the immune system, and include substances such as interferons, transfer factor, levamisole, and gamma globulins. Interferon-α has been shown to have a weak benefit in MS, and its use is associated with unpleasant side-effects. The use of interferon-β has so far been reported only by intraspinal injection; a controlled trial of interferon-β used in this way has shown a moderate decrease in exacerbations. Further studies are needed to confirm this effect, and to test whether it may not be equally useful by simpler routes of administration.

Interferon-γ seems to worsen MS, and, in the opinion of the Committee, its use should be avoided. The effects of transfer factor are equivocal but mostly negative, and the reported results of levamisole treatment are conflicting: levamisole requires further study. Gamma globulin injections are probably ineffective; monoclonal antibody treatment is interesting, but there are no developments of practical usefulness yet.

Plasmapheresis and lymphocytapheresis are expensive physical means of removing blood plasma and lymphocytes, respectively. Difficult controlled studies of plasmapheresis have been reported. Some have shown no benefit, but others have shown improvement and reduction in the frequency of the attacks. Most such efforts have employed combined therapy with azathioprine and/or prednisone as well. The rationale of plasmapheresis is to remove antibodies thought to be responsible for MS; no antibodies shown to be specific for MS have been described, however. Because of this and the expense of the procedure, there is still no consensus in the neurological community that plasmapheresis is useful.

Large controlled studies of lymphocytapheresis, the physical removal of large numbers of lymphocytes from the blood, have not been done. Several small studies have shown conflicting results; because of this the procedure cannot be recommended now except in controlled trials. Lymphocytapheresis is a very expensive mode of treatment.

One controlled trial of total lymphoid irradiation, the removal of many lymphocytes by radiation treatment, has shown promising results in chronic progressive MS. Although the method is not without risk, it is fairly well tolerated, and has a long history of use in other diseases; the long-term hazards, occurring in only a small percentage of patients, are known. The method deserves more clinical trials in progressive MS.

Various combinations of immunosuppressive drugs and procedures are commonly used; for example, plasmapheresis and lymphocytapheresis are often used in combination with other immunosuppressive drugs such as prednisone, azathioprine, or cyclophosphamide. Such combinations are used with the aim of increasing effectiveness, and at the same time decreasing toxicity of individual agents. None of these regimens has been demonstrated to be effective in controlled trials, in the opinion of the Committee. All are expensive and carry considerable risk.

Desensitization treatment has been used by repeatedly injecting MBP from animals into patients; this trial was a failure. A synthetic analog of MBP, the four-aminoacid peptide COP-I, has been used in similar attempts, and both pilot and controlled studies have shown good results in reducing the frequency of exacerbations of MS. Most workers agree, however, that further studies of COP-I, involving larger numbers of patients, must be done. Unfortunately, the supply of COP-I is currently very small and additional studies have not been possible to date.

Currently there is more interest in antiviral drugs as potential modifiers of the MS process. Some of this interest derives from recent evidence that common viral infections seem to be the chief risk factors in triggering new attacks of the illness. The reported effectiveness of both interferon-α and -β in reducing the exacerbation rate might be explained by reduction or modification of such infections. Both herpes simplex and herpes zoster are potential candidates for viral triggering of attacks, and this has stimulated interest in the possibility of using acyclovir, an effective antiherpes agent, in future MS treatment trials. Amantadine, a drug effective in preventing and treating influenza type A infections, has shown no effect in short pilot trials, but deserves further study; more trials of methisoprinol, another agent with antiviral properties, are also planned on the basis of encouraging but inconclusive pilot studies.

Other miscellaneous methods are also discussed in this chapter.

THE IMMUNE SYSTEM AND MULTIPLE SCLEROSIS

A brief review of the immune system is important, because current theories favor the idea that MS is an immunologic disease. The normal function of the immune system is to recognize and repel foreign invaders, such as bacteria, viruses, and other foreign substances *(antigens)*. Normally it is careful to recognize "self" components, and not destroy these by mistake.

Almost 60 years ago it was shown that repeated injections of brain extracts in animals would make a few of them develop an inflammatory disease of the CNS called *experimental allergic encephalomyelitis (EAE)*. By injection of myelin or certain proteins contained in myelin—e.g., MBP or proteolipid protein (PLP)—with killed tuberculosis organisms and paraffin oil, a maximal immunologic attack on the CNS could be caused in certain species of rats, mice, guinea pigs, and monkeys. EAE was quite similar to a disease accidentally produced in some humans with an old preparation of rabies vaccine that contained fragments of myelin. *Postrabies vaccine encephalomyelitis,* in turn, was quite similar pathologically to occasional forms of *postinfectious encephalomyelitis* appearing in a few unlucky children after naturally occurring measles, rubella, chickenpox, and—occasionally—other viruses. Postinfectious encephalomyelitis in humans is not a recurrent disease, and only happens once. It has been shown recently that children develop T-lymphocytes immunized against MBP prior to development of postmeasles encephalomyelitis. Later, it was shown that a chronic relapsing form of EAE could be produced in some genetically susceptible animals by the inoculation of young animals. These animals recovered from attacks of paralysis, only to develop symptoms weeks or months later, in a manner similar to MS. Moreover, pathological changes in the CNS in such animals are much like those seen in MS. This has been the strongest reason for *many to assume that MS is an "autoim-*

mune" *disease*, one in which the immune system, for some reason, has turned against its own CNS.

Although this remains an attractive theory, there are some important differences between MS and chronic EAE. Antibodies to myelin proteins are difficult to find in the blood of MS patients, in contrast to EAE. Anti-MBP antibodies have been found in the spinal fluid of MS patients, but it is not yet clear if they contribute to the illness, or are a consequence of it. In EAE the antigen is clearly myelin or a myelin component; in MS the antigen is still unknown. Another important difference is that EAE is easily inhibited and suppressed by a number of drugs that seem to have little benefit for MS patients.

The immune system is complex. Its basic units are two kinds of white blood cells located in the thymus, spleen, and lymph nodes. These circulate, by way of the blood and lymph, to all parts of the body. The larger cells are *macrophages* (Greek: "big-eaters"). They function by engulfing and disposing of debris; they also secrete chemicals known as proteases, one of which—plasminogen activator—is capable of causing destruction of myelin. Other chemicals produced by macrophages are prostaglandins: some of these promote inflammation and immune functions, whereas others suppress the same functions.

The smaller cells are lymphocytes, which come in several varieties. B-lymphocytes are processed in the bone marrow and become antibody-producing cells. The more numerous T-lymphocytes are mostly processed in the thymus gland and can be divided into several classes, the more important being T-helper, T-suppressor, and T-killer cells. T-lymphocytes become *activated* when exposed to an antigen to which they are reactive; the cell becomes metabolically more active, enlarges, and secretes a group of chemicals called *lymphokines;* some of the functions of lymphokines are to promote enlargement of lymphocyte populations, activate macrophages, increase blood flow and edema of tissue, and attract other types of white blood cells to the area. Interferon-γ is one such lymphokine secreted by activated T-cells; it is a substance that facilitates antigen recognition; its use in treatment has been associated with a marked increase in the frequency of MS exacerbations.

Several laboratories have shown that T-suppressor activity is decreased in the blood early in a new exacerbation of MS. The exact significance of this is unknown, but it may be a factor in accounting for evidence of an unusually active immune system in MS patients (see page 10: Who Gets Multiple Sclerosis?). Lymphocytes in the CSF in MS are mostly T-lymphocytes, and their number and the relative number of T-helper cells increases with attacks.

Many B-lymphocytes also exist in and around the MS plaques, but they are relatively uncommon in the CSF; they are the source of local immunoglobulin production. Immunoglobulins are usually antibodies, but in the case of MS the antigen is unknown, and efforts to find the antigen by studying the antibodies have been largely unsuccessful so far.

IMMUNE SYSTEM: IMMUNOSUPPRESSION

Azathioprine (Imuran)

Description: Azathioprine is an immunosuppressive drug in wide use for the past 20 years. It is a synthetic chemical compound.

Rationale: Azathioprine belongs to a group of drugs that modify nucleic acid or protein metabolism of cells, known as anti-metabolites, and that exert a potent suppressive effect on the immune system. It is very effective in suppression of EAE, a possible animal model of MS.

Evaluation: Several controlled trials with azathioprine have been completed. Two have shown little difference between drug-treated and placebo-treated patients, but three other studies agree that azathioprine slows the progression of disability, even though the frequency of exacerbations may not be changed. The drug is widely used in the United States, but more so in Europe where it has been reported that the effect in arresting progression is most evident after 5–10 years. The results of a new United Kingdom trial are awaited with interest.

Azathioprine is now being used frequently in combination with other agents, such as ACTH, steroids, plasmapheresis, etc.

Risks/Costs: There are risks, including depression of bone marrow, especially the white blood cells; changes in liver function; skin rashes, and infection due to depression of immune defenses. A major concern is a modest increase in the frequency of cancer, chiefly non-Hodgkin's lymphoma. In one group of patients with rheumatoid arthritis and other disorders treated for up to 10 years, among 1,109 patients 40 cases of cancer developed, compared with an expected rate of 28.6 in the general population. Some patients cannot tolerate the drug due to nausea.

Conclusion: At the present time, evidence suggests that azathioprine is suitable for use in patients with increasing deficit from MS, where the risks of therapy may be less than risks of severe disability. The results of recently completed trials are awaited, however. Careful monitoring of the patient and blood tests are necessary throughout the course of treatment.

In the opinion of the Committee, this therapy has been demonstrated to have limited usefulness in selected patients. Its use carries significant risk.

IMMUNE SYSTEM: IMMUNOSUPPRESSION

Cyclophosphamide (Cytoxan)

Description: Cyclophosphamide is an alkylating agent developed in connection with cancer treatment programs. It interferes with the metabolism of cells, especially rapidly dividing cells such as white blood cells, and hair follicles. It kills lymphocytes and thus induces immunosuppression, and promotes the development of tolerance to various antigens. It is very effective in suppressing EAE, a possible animal model of MS.

Evaluation: Cyclophosphamide has been used in MS treatment for many years; its early use was mostly in uncontrolled studies, where it was often, but not always, reported to improve the condition of patients with chronic progressive MS, especially those having only modest disability (DSS score less than 5) at the beginning of treatment. Later a controlled U.S. study treated 20 progressive MS patients with high-dose cyclophosphamide and ACTH, 20 with ACTH alone, and 18 with plasmapheresis and low-dose cyclophosphamide, and reported that 80% of the first group were stable at 1 year, compared with 20% of the second group and 50% of the plasmapheresis group. A more recent study from California, however, found no difference between cyclophosphamide-treated and placebo-treated patients when the evaluating physician was "blinded" by doing the repeat evaluation only after the regrowth of hair (always lost with high-dose treatment).

Risks/Costs: Short-term treatment with high doses produces hair loss, nausea, occasional bladder injury, and risk of infection; long-term risks include sterility, mutations, and increased risk of cancer.

Conclusion: The conflicting reports about the usefulness of this drug warrant caution in its use, in view of the potentially serious and unpleasant side-effects reported. Greater experience with more patients in continuing clinical trials should clarify whether it has a place in the treatment of MS.

In the opinion of the Committee, this therapy may have some efficacy, but the evidence is conflicting, and it must be regarded as investigational. Its use carries significant risk.

IMMUNE SYSTEM: IMMUNOSUPPRESSION

Cyclosporine A

Description: This drug is a simple peptide molecule (a chain of 11 aminoacids) isolated from certain fungal extracts.

Rationale: Cyclosporine A is an effective immunosuppressive agent, the drug chiefly responsible for the current high rate of success with kidney, heart, and liver transplants. It acts by selectively inhibiting helper T-lymphocytes and killer T-lymphocytes. It has been found to be effective in many cases of uveitis, an inflammatory disease of the eye. Uveitis occurs most commonly as an independent illness, but also is seen in 5–15% of MS patients. The agent has had some limited effectiveness in the animal disease, EAE.

Evaluation: Pilot studies in Canada and Europe showed that cyclosporine A does not prevent exacerbations and halt progression in all cases of MS. A recently reported study from Germany compared cyclosporine A and azathioprine treatment results in 167 patients: No clear benefit from cyclosporine A could be shown in comparison with azathioprine. The preliminary results of a cooperative U.S. study in more than 400 patients showed a statistically significant slowing of progression, in comparison with placebo-treated patients, but the data analysis at the time of this publication is incomplete: the exact extent of the benefit and whether it is sufficient to justify the risk of chronic therapy is presently unknown. The results of a joint United Kingdom–Dutch trial of cyclosporine A likewise indicate some benefit, but full analysis of results will be necessary to know if the benefits outweighed the risks.

Risks/Costs: In most cases cyclosporine A produces some impairment of kidney function, which produces no symptoms and is usually reversible when the drug is discontinued. Some permanent microscopic changes may persist, however. Gum and hair overgrowth and variable degrees of high blood pressure are the other main side-effects. Used alone, it does not seem to lead to increased cancer rates, although cancer rates in transplant patients are generally increased.

Conclusions: Because of its costs and side-effects, the drug cannot be recommended now for use outside of a clinical trial—at least until the full results of recent large clinical trials become available in the near future.

In the opinion of the Committee, this therapy may have some efficacy, but the evidence is conflicting, and it must be regarded as investigational. Long-term use may be associated with significant serious side-effects.

IMMUNE SYSTEM: IMMUNOSUPPRESSION

Antilymphocyte Serum, Antilymphocyte Globulin

Description: Antilymphocyte serum (ALS) is prepared by immunizing horses with injections of human lymphocytes from spleen, thymus, and/or peripheral blood to produce antibodies against lymphocytes. The serum or purified antibody containing globulins from this blood is injected into patients.

Rationale: Injection of ALS or ALG is very effective in destroying lymphocytes in the circulation, and thus is highly immunosuppressive. Most reports use regimens of ALS or ALG at the beginning of a treatment program that also includes ACTH, prednisone, or other corticosteroids. Frequently azathioprine is then continued on a long-term basis to maintain some immunosuppressive effect.

Evaluation: Most reports deal with regimens of ALS or ALG used in combination with other immunosuppressive drugs, such as azathioprine or cyclophosphamide. Because ALS or ALG is used typically for only a brief period, it is difficult to separate its effect from the effect of these drugs. ALS and ALG have not been used alone.

Risks/Costs: Adverse reactions include local inflammatory reactions, rash, hives, fever, lymph node enlargement, and purpura (bleeding tendency). Many of these are allergic reactions to horse serum. Patients known to be sensitive have usually been excluded.

Conclusion: ALS and ALG are not now suitable for general use. They may be used as part of a larger immunosuppressive program by those familiar with their risks and toxic effects. Used in this way they certainly contribute to immunosuppression.

In the opinion of the Committee, this therapy may have some efficacy, but the evidence is conflicting, and it must be regarded as investigational. Its use carries significant risk.

IMMUNE SYSTEM: IMMUNOSUPPRESSION

Antilymphocyte Monoclonal Antibodies: Mouse Monoclonal Antibodies, Human Monoclonal Antibodies

Description: Advances in biotechnology in the past 12 years have made it possible to produce in the laboratory large amounts of single (monoclonal) antibodies in tissue culture. Thus it is now possible to produce antibodies reacting with certain lymphocyte types or with certain receptors on the cell membranes of lymphocytes. Theoretically, this should make it possible to augment or suppress immune responses with less risk than heretofore possible with drugs and other methods.

Monoclonal antibodies have so far been used primarily in diagnosis of various viral and bacterial diseases, and in other aspects of laboratory research. Treatment attempts to date (in cancer, organ transplants, and many other illnesses, including MS) have mostly been made with mouse monoclonal antibodies (MMAbs), and these have had only limited success, in large part due to the fact that many patients make antibodies that neutralize the MMAbs. Human monoclonal antibodies (HuMAbs) can now be made, which may circumvent this problem, but so far not in the amounts necessary for large treatment trials.

Rationale: The rationale is the same as for the use of ALS or ALG. However, although ALS or ALG might be likened to shotguns, monoclonal antibodies are more like rifles—able to hit very selective targets.

Evaluation: Preliminary studies were done in 15 MS patients using MMAbs against human T-lymphocytes. There was a transient disappearance of T-lymphocytes from the blood; however, the duration of the study was too short to evaluate the effect on the MS. Future studies are planned using monoclonal antibodies against major histocompatibility complexes.

Risks/Costs: Allergic reactions may occur in response to injection of foreign serum. All of these therapies will be expensive.

Conclusion: Monoclonal antibody therapy theoretically offers much promise in the future, especially when it will be possible with HuMAbs. At the moment, however, the treatment is not available except in a few trials, and it is too early to judge what the effects will be.

In the opinion of the Committee, the rationale of this therapy is plausible, but the results of controlled trials are not yet available, and it must be regarded as investigational. Its use carries significant risk. It is very expensive.

IMMUNE SYSTEM: IMMUNOSUPPRESSION

Total Lymphoid Irradiation

Description: Over a 5–6 week period lymph nodes over the entire body are irradiated with x-rays, in small daily doses, in an attempt to destroy most existing lymphoid tissue. Vital organs, such as the heart, bone marrow, spinal cord, etc., are carefully shielded from the x-rays.

Rationale: Lymphocytes and their products are the mediators of tissue destruction in autoimmune diseases. Total lymphoid irradiation (TLI) has a record of producing prolonged immunosuppression and sustained relief in a number of patients with rheumatoid arthritis. The reduction in lymphocytes is very long-lasting.

Evaluation: One study of the effects of TLI in MS has been reported. During a 21-month follow-up period, 20 patients receiving TLI had less worsening of their disease than did a control group of 20 patients. Patients with higher lymphocyte counts generally did worse: a follow-up study in the same patients showed that those maintaining a total lymphocyte count of 900/mm^3 or less had less progression of MS over a 2-year period.

Risks/Costs: Costs are high. TLI has a long record of use in many thousands of patients with Hodgkin's disease during the past 30 years, and generally it has a good record of safety, and the risks are well known in such patients. There is apparently a low risk of cancer, lower than would be expected with conventional immunosuppressive drugs. During treatment, fatigue, nausea, transient hair loss, dry mouth, and skin irritations may occur, but such symptoms usually subside in 2 months. Other reported complications are shingles (herpes zoster) and transient pericarditis.

Conclusion: The method needs further study, but appears promising for use in patients with rapidly worsening disability, because of relatively low risk and the results reported to date. Larger controlled trials will be necessary before the method can be recommended for general use; such studies are now in progress. Information is also needed from longer follow-up of patients already treated by TLI.

In the opinion of the Committee, the rationale of this therapy is plausible, but the results of controlled trials are not yet available, and it must be regarded as investigational. Its use carries significant risk. It is very expensive.

IMMUNE SYSTEM: IMMUNOSUPPRESSION

Thoracic Duct Drainage

Description: The thoracic duct is the major lymphatic vessel, receiving lymph containing many lymphocytes from most of the body. A tube is placed in the thoracic duct in the neck to drain off and discard lymphatic fluid.

Rationale: Thoracic duct drainage (TDD) markedly reduces lymphocyte counts and thus suppresses immune reactivity.

Evaluation: In one study TDD was done in five patients for from 6–23 days. There were no controls. The results were inconclusive.

Risks/Costs: The risks are those associated with general surgery, and those associated with severe immunosuppression: infections and cancer. Prolonged use is hard on the patient and carries the additional risk of lymphatic obstruction. It is a very expensive treatment.

Conclusion: This is an expensive and risky procedure that has no clear-cut advantages over other techniques of immunosuppression such as TLI and the use of immunosuppressive drugs.

In the opinion of the Committee, the rationale of this therapy is plausible, but the results of controlled trials are not yet available, and it must be regarded as investigational. Its use carries significant risk. It is very expensive.

IMMUNE SYSTEM: IMMUNOSUPPRESSION

Plasmapheresis (Plasma Exchange)

Description: Blood is removed from the patient, and the liquid plasma and the cells are separated by centrifuge. The plasma (including many lymphocytes) is discarded and replaced by normal plasma or human albumin to avoid loss of protein and fluid. The "reconstituted" blood is then returned to the patient's circulation. The process is repeated a number of times at intervals.

Rationale: Substances have been described in the plasma of MS patients that can damage myelin and/or impair nerve conduction. Such substances are not specific to MS, however, and may be seen in some normals, as well as in other diseases. When they occur in MS, it is not clear that they are important in the production of plaques; however, if they are important in causing the disease, or producing loss of nerve conduction, removal might cause improvement.

Evaluation: There are numerous reports of the use of plasmapheresis on small numbers of patients in uncontrolled trials. Almost all studies have used plasmapheresis in conjunction with other immunosuppressive drugs. An early controlled study found that patients with slowly progressive MS receiving plasma exchange (PE) and azathioprine did no better than those receiving azathioprine alone. In another controlled study, however, patients receiving PE plus low-dose cyclophosphamide plus alternate-day prednisone did better than patients treated with sham PE plus these drugs—by some methods of statistical analysis, but not by others. Additional controlled studies are now under way in the United States and Canada.

Risks/Costs: PE is expensive, costing more than $500 per treatment for each exchange, and the procedure is usually repeated every few days or weeks. Risks include fainting during the procedure, and a reduction in red blood cells and platelets with repeated use.

Conclusion: The value of PE has yet to be proven in the treatment of MS. Controlled studies done to date are not convincing, and, in view of its high cost, the procedure should remain investigative until the results of other studies are available.

In the opinion of the Committee, this therapy may have some efficacy, but the evidence is conflicting, and it must be regarded as investigational. It is relatively free of serious adverse side-effects during long-term use. It is very expensive.

IMMUNE SYSTEM: IMMUNOSUPPRESSION

Lymphocytapheresis (Leukapheresis)

Description: Lymphocytapheresis is a procedure in which blood is withdrawn from the patient, and most of the lymphocytes removed and discarded; the remaining white blood cells, red blood cells, and plasma are returned to the patient. The procedure is automated and requires about 2 h.

Rationale: Lymphocytes are necessary to mediate most autoimmune diseases; the procedure is designed to remove significant numbers of lymphocytes with the presumption that MS is an autoimmune disease.

Evaluation: Several uncontrolled trials of lymphocytapheresis have been reported with variable results. In one clinic patients were thought to be improved to a greater extent than might have been expected spontaneously. Three other small trials showed no benefit from the procedure, and five centers reported inconclusive results in small trials. In the largest study of 70 patients, positive effects were claimed in relapsing–remitting as well as in chronic progressive MS, but almost half of the patients discontinued the treatment before the end of the study.

Risks/Costs: Lymphocytapheresis is very expensive, and has to be repeated frequently if any significant reduction in lymphocyte population is to be achieved. Blood platelets are modestly reduced in most patients during treatment (approximately 25% reduction). Most studies have been short-term, and the long-term results of treatment remain unknown.

Conclusion: The benefits of lymphocytapheresis are unproven, in the absence of a controlled study. Because of this, very high costs, and possible long-term risks, lymphocytapheresis is not recommended as a treatment for MS, except in the setting of a clinical trial.

In the opinion of the Committee, the rationale of this therapy is plausible, but it has not been adequately tested, and must be regarded as experimental. Long-term use may be associated with significant serious side-effects. It is very expensive.

IMMUNE SYSTEM: IMMUNOSUPPRESSION

Methotrexate

Description: This is a synthetic immunosuppressive drug, taken orally or by injection.

Rationale: Methotrexate is a folic acid antagonist; it inhibits DNA synthesis and cell division and is both immunosuppressive and an effective anticancer agent. At low dose, it is a highly effective short-term treatment for the inflammatory joint lesions of rheumatoid arthritis, an "autoimmune disease." Its effect is greatest in patients carrying the genetic marker HLA-DR2, which is present in approximately half of MS patients. Its potential usefulness in MS is emphasized by the fact that it effectively prevents EAE, a model disease resembling MS, in several species of laboratory animal.

Evaluation: Methotrexate was tested in a single double-blind trial in MS in the early 1970s and interest has lapsed since then. Twenty-seven patients were treated with methotrexate (alternating with 6-mercaptopurine, a related immunosuppressive agent) or placebo. There was no sign of improvement, as compared with the placebo group, over a total observation period of 10–23 months.

Risks/Costs: Treatment is inexpensive. The most common side-effect is mucosal irritation, sometimes progressing to frank ulceration, with an assortment of gastrointestinal symptoms. Chemical hepatitis, lasting a week or more, occurs in approximately one-fifth of methotrexate-treated patients and progresses occasionally to hepatic fibrosis or cirrhosis. Factors predisposing to fibrosis (obesity, diabetes, excessive alcohol intake) should be contraindications to its use. Whether there is a long-term danger of cancer is uncertain.

Conclusion: The results of reported treatment do not justify further use of methotrexate in MS.

In the opinion of the Committee, this therapy has been adequately tested and shown to be without value. Its use carries significant risk.

IMMUNE SYSTEM: IMMUNOSUPPRESSION

Chlorambucil (Leukeran)

Description: Another alkylating agent used in cancer chemo-therapy and resembling cyclophosphamide in its action.

Rationale: This drug is used in treating lymphomas and leukemias. The justification for its use is the same as for preceding drugs in this section.

Evaluation: In a small open trial carried out in Ireland, MS patients treated with chlorambucil were compared with similar patients given a placebo. The results were comparable to those obtained with other immunosuppressive agents.

Risks/Costs: Side-effects are like those of other powerful cancer drugs: nausea and vomiting, bone marrow depression, temporary suppression of fertility, and intercurrent infections. These are all rapidly reversible unless the drug is continued for a long period. Late cancer due to the drug is an unassessed possibility.

Conclusion: This treatment is not recommended.

In the opinion of the Committee, there appears to be no generally accepted scientific basis for use of this therapy. It has never been tested in a proper controlled trial. Its use carries significant risk.

IMMUNE SYSTEM: IMMUNOSUPPRESSION

1-(2-Chloroethyl)-3-Cyclohexyl-1-Nitrosourea (Lomustine), 5-Fluorouracil

Description: Lomustine (CCNU) is an alkylating agent and 5-fluorouracil (5-FU) an antimetabolite, both used in cancer chemotherapy and resembling cyclophosphamide in many of their properties. CCNU is given orally and 5-FU intravenously.

Rationale: It is the same as for cyclophosphamide. CCNU is of particular interest because it penetrates the CNS much more efficiently than cyclophosphamide or 5-FU.

Evaluation: Preliminary trials of the two drugs have been carried out in small groups of patients with progressive or stabilized MS given a single course of treatment. Although treatment, in each case, produced significant change in cellular and other immunological characteristics, it did not affect the course of disease.

Risks/Costs: The long-term risk of leukemia is high. Short-term effects include nausea and vomiting, fever, and thrombocytopenia or leukopenia.

Conclusion: These drugs are not recommended for use in MS.

In the opinion of the Committee, this therapy should not be used because of reported harmful effects.

IMMUNE SYSTEM: IMMUNOSUPPRESSION

Mitoxantrone (Novatrone)

Description: An anthracenedione derivative that is widely used for treatment of breast cancer and certain leukemias. It is administered intravenously, in a short course of daily infusions.

Rationale: This drug belongs to another class of cancer chemotherapy agents with immunosuppressive properties. Its efficacy is greatly enhanced when it is used together with cytosine arabinoside. It has proved highly effective in suppressing the animal model disease, EAE.

Evaluation: Clinical trials in MS are in the planning stage.

Risks/Costs: Mitoxantrone shows considerably less acute toxicity (nausea, vomiting, loss of hair) than other cancer drugs of comparable potency. The most serious side-effect, seen in 3–4% of treated patients, is cardiotoxicity. Lesser problems are prolonged depression of the circulating white cells and platelets.

Conclusion: There are as yet no reports of the effects of this drug in MS.

In the opinion of the Committee, the rationale of this therapy is plausible, but it has not been adequately tested, and must be regarded as experimental. Its use carries significant risk.

IMMUNE SYSTEM: IMMUNE MODULATION

Levamisole

Description: Levamisole is a synthetic drug originally used, and still used, to treat certain roundworm infections of the intestinal tract. It has been found to have positive effects on the immune system by restoring defective T-cell function.

Rationale: T-suppressor cells are present in decreased numbers early in MS attacks; one theory of autoimmune disease attributes the disease to such suppressor-cell deficiency, allowing uncontrolled T-helper lymphocytes to react in an abnormal fashion to "self" antigens. Therefore, the use of levamisole as an immunostimulant in MS appeared to be worthy of trial.

Evaluation: Early studies with levamisole in small numbers of patients suggested that the drug might worsen the disease. A much larger double-blind trial in 85 patients in Belgium denies this effect, however, and rather showed a modest benefit in the treated patients, with some slowing of progression.

Risks/Costs: The drug was well tolerated in the largest trial, although one patient had a low white blood cell count, possibly due to the drug, which caused no symptoms. Cost is moderate.

Conclusion: Present evidence suggests that levamisole may be safe in MS, but the beneficial results reported in the largest trial were not strong enough to be statistically significant. Further trials with this agent are needed and at least one is planned in Italy. At the moment, the question of usefulness cannot be answered conclusively.

In the opinion of the Committee, this therapy may have some efficacy, but the evidence is conflicting, and it must be regarded as investigational. It is relatively free of serious adverse side-effects during short-term use.

IMMUNE SYSTEM: IMMUNE MODULATION

Colchicine

Description: A complex chemical (alkaloid) originally known as an extract of *Colchicum* (the crocus flower). An old drug that has been in use for more than 200 years, it is used most commonly for the treatment of acute gout, but more recently has been found to have not only antiinflammatory but also immunosuppressive properties.

Rationale: Colchicine reduced the numbers of T-helper and T-suppressor cells in normal human volunteers; it is also effective in suppressing EAE in animals. Among its actions are the ability to enhance prostaglandin production, and to inhibit macrophage functions.

Evaluation: Encouraging findings in a small pilot study in MS patients led to a double-blind controlled trial in chronic progressive MS, which is still in progress in New York.

Risks/Costs: Colchicine is an inexpensive drug. It may cause side-effects such as nausea, vomiting, diarrhea, and abdominal pain. Less commonly it can produce serious side-effects such as peripheral neuritis, muscle disease, and bone marrow toxicity, and long-term safety is thus questionable.

Conclusion: The drug is not currently recommended for general use; the results of the current trials are not yet available.

In the opinion of the Committee, the rationale of this therapy is plausible, but the results of controlled trials are not yet available, and it must be regarded as investigational. Long-term use may be associated with significant serious side-effects.

IMMUNE SYSTEM: IMMUNE MODULATION

Danazol (Danocrine)

Description: Danazol is a synthetic androgen (male hormone) that has minimal virilizing effects.

Rationale: Danazol has been used primarily in the treatment of endometriosis and cystic disease of the breast. However, it also has immune modulating properties. For example, it decreases platelet antibodies in idiopathic thrombocytopenic purpura, and is often effective in that autoimmune disorder. It has also been used in the treatment of urticaria (hives), and in the treatment of hereditary angioedema very effectively.

Evaluation: There are, as yet, no reports on the use of danazol in MS. However, one trial is under way, in view of the effectiveness of this agent in other immune disorders.

Risks/Costs: Costs are moderate. Danazol must not be used during pregnancy or in patients with known liver disease. The reported side-effects are mainly those common to male hormone: mild masculinizing effects, oily skin, acne, weight gain. Prominent psychological effects have been reported.

Conclusion: The results of the current trial are awaited. No information on the use of danazol in MS is yet available.

In the opinion of the Committee, the rationale of this therapy is plausible, but the results of controlled trials are not yet available, and it must be regarded as investigational. It is relatively free of serious adverse side-effects during short-term use. Long-term use may be associated with significant serious side-effects.

IMMUNE SYSTEM: IMMUNE MODULATION

Thymus Hormones: Thymosin, Thymuline (Facteur Thymique Serique), Thymopentin (Thymopoietin 5), TFX-Polfa, THX, T-Aktivin

Description: Protein hormones, extracted from calf thymus, or biologically active fragments of these hormones. Many of these are now available as synthetic compounds.

Rationale: Approximately 15 hormone-like compounds have been isolated from calf thymus (or from the circulating blood) and many if not all of them act on T-lymphocytes and modulate immune reactions. They are being actively tested in autoimmune diseases such as rheumatoid arthritis as well as in immunodeficiencies and cancer. In a limited experiment, thymosin failed to suppress EAE, the model disease, in guinea pigs. However, because MS patients present abnormalities in immunoregulatory subsets of T-cells, it appears possible that thymosin or other natural hormones or synthetic copies of these might correct abnormalities.

Evaluation: In three pilot studies, relapses were not affected and there was little or no effect on chronic progression. In one trial, TFX-Polfa was used alternately with nitrogen mustard and levamisole, and benefit was said to result in 80% of treated patients. Several controlled trials are now in progress: thymosin (fraction 5) in the U.S., thymuline (a synthetic 9 amino acid peptide) in France, and TFX-Polfa in Poland.

T-aktivin has been advocated as a cure for a variety of diseases, including MS, tumors, psoriasis, sarcoidosis, even blood poisoning, but no controlled studies of this material have been reported. Similarly, THX, which is essentially a crude, nonsterile extract of calf thymus, has also been publicized widely as an effective treatment for a variety of unrelated chronic ailments, including MS. This material was responsible for several documented cases of sepsis (overwhelming infection) in treated patients.

Risks/Costs: None known for most of these products. THX is nonsterile and produces infections in patients who receive it.

Conclusion: Based on the evidence examined by the Committee, this treatment is not recommended at the present time.

In the opinion of the Committee, there appears to be no generally accepted scientific basis for use of this therapy. It has never been tested in a proper controlled trial. Its use carries significant risk.

IMMUNE SYSTEM: IMMUNE MODULATION

Thymectomy

Description: Surgical removal of the thymus gland from the upper chest.

Rationale: T-lymphocytes are processed by the thymus gland, some even in later life. Thymectomy is very effective treatment in myasthenia gravis, a known autoimmune disease, especially in children and young adults.

Evaluation: One study of 34 patients from St. Louis showed that thymectomy did not benefit patients with MS. Patients with relapsing–remitting and chronic progressive types of MS were treated: neither group did better than controls, and the progressive group did slightly worse with thymectomy.

Conclusion: Thymectomy has been demonstrated to have no benefit, and further trials of this method are not recommended.

In the opinion of the Committee, this therapy has been adequately tested and shown to be without value.

Transfer Factor

Description: Transfer factor (TF) is a substance extracted from disrupted blood lymphocytes that can transfer, when injected into another individual, cell-mediated immunity to viruses or other antigens to which the donor is immune. It is prepared in an experimental laboratory by nonstandardized procedures, and the preparation is laborious and expensive. It is not available commercially.

Rationale: If MS is due to defective immunity, or if it is due to a persistent virus, TF might enhance MS patients' resistance to MS.

Evaluation: Three controlled trials using TF for 6–13 months produced negative results. In one trial, 30 patients receiving TF were compared with 30 control MS patients; there was slightly less progression in the treated group, but results were not apparent for 18 months, and benefit was apparent only in patients with mild disability. Exacerbation rate was not affected. In another study, 70 patients receiving TF were compared with 35 patients receiving placebo: there were no differences between the groups at 36 months. A more recent Australian trial of TF has also shown no effect.

Risks/Costs: The cost is high; risks are low.

Conclusion: TF as used in reported studies is of no benefit to MS patients. Problems in standardization of TF and the expense of preparation, when considered in the light of published results, make it unlikely that this form of therapy deserves further consideration.

In the opinion of the Committee, this therapy has been adequately tested and shown to be without value. It is relatively free of serious adverse side-effects during long-term use.

IMMUNE SYSTEM: IMMUNE MODULATION

Transfer of Lymphocytes

Description: Transfer of blood lymphocytes from healthy individuals to human-leukocyte-antigen-compatible patients with MS. Donor lymphocytes are obtained by leukapheresis and administered intravenously to the recipient.

Rationale: There are indications that MS may result from a deficiency of specific or nonspecific suppressor T-lymphocyte activity. In identical twin pairs discordant for MS, the healthy twin is presumed to resist the disease process by an adequate suppressor T-cell response and the MS twin to fail because of lack of these cells. Transfer of these cells should correct the deficiency in the MS twin.

Evaluation: A preliminary trial is under way in the United States in a small series of identical twin pairs. Approximately three billion lymphocytes are transferred from the healthy twin to the MS twin in each case. If the result of this trial is suggestive, the procedure may be extended to nonidentical donor–recipient pairs.

Risks/Costs: No untoward effects were observed in the first patients transfused. In recipients of lymphocytes from nonidentical donors, a number of serious immunologic complications may or may not occur. The procedure is very expensive.

Conclusion: The results of current trials are awaited with interest.

In the opinion of the Committee, the rationale of this therapy is plausible, but the results of controlled trials are not yet available, and it must be regarded as investigational. Its use carries significant risk.

IMMUNE SYSTEM: DESENSITIZATION OR SPECIFIC IMMUNE TOLERANCE

Myelin Basic Protein

Description: A protein extracted from pig or cattle brain, injected under the skin (subcutaneously) in repeated doses.

Rationale: MBP is the protein component of myelin that is effective in producing the autoimmune disease EAE in experimental animals. Large repeated doses of MBP can prevent or suppress the development of EAE in such animals.

Evaluation: Several small, uncontrolled trials of MBP in the treatment of MS have been carried out. In the most thorough trial to date, a group of patients received daily injections of large, increasing doses of porcine MBP over a 2-year period. However, new bouts and continued progression were observed in most treated patients. Two of eight patients with progressive MS showed an amount of improvement that was unexpected, raising the possibility that a subset of MS patients may be benefited by MBP.

Risks/Costs: Side-effects included actual immunization of the patients by the injection procedure, as shown by local delayed hypersensitivity reactions at the injection site; there was also temporary worsening of neurologic symptoms and signs after some injections in some patients. At present, the risks would be judged to outweigh the limited possible benefit. Costs at present are high.

Conclusion: On the basis of trials that have been done, this treatment should not be regarded as effective.

In the opinion of the Committee, this therapy has been adequately tested and shown to be without value. Its use carries significant risk.

IMMUNE SYSTEM: DESENSITIZATION

Copolymer I

Description: COP-I is a synthetic chain of four amino acids, an analog of the MBP molecule, which does not produce EAE when injected into animals or humans; it protects animals against EAE. It is given in repeated doses subcutaneously.

Rationale: MBP causes EAE and has long been suspected of being the MS antigen, but without adequate proof. MBP is probably the antigen responsible for the allergic reaction in the brain in post-infectious encephalomyelitis (see page 50: The Immune System and Multiple Sclerosis). Repeated injections of MBP are risky and have been shown to be ineffective in MS treatment. COP-I was tried because it could protect animals against EAE, in the hope that it could also stop the progress of MS.

Evaluation: Early uncontrolled studies were positive. Recently, in a controlled trial 25 patients received COP-I daily and were compared with 23 patients who received placebo injections daily. There were 62 exacerbations in the placebo group and only 16 in the COP-I group. Mildly disabled patients worsened by .5 DSS units in 2 years when they received COP-I, and by 1.2 DSS units in 2 years in the placebo group. There was some difficulty in maintaining double-blind conditions, because COP-I caused itching, soreness, and redness of the arm at injection sites in most patients.

Risks/Costs: Costs are estimated to be high when the drug is available. Risks were slight in the trial reported: sore arms at injection sites; occasional general allergic reactions (anaphylactoid): anxiety, flushing, dizziness, and difficulty breathing— passing in 5–15 min after injection.

Conclusions: The authors of the successful trial in exacerbating-remitting cases cited believe that further confirmatory trials are necessary in a larger number of patients, and the Committee agrees with this assessment. Unfortunately, the drug is not available now, which will delay new studies. Alternative similar peptides are being studied in animals and may become available for clinical trials.

In the opinion of the Committee, the rationale of this therapy is plausible, but it has not been adequately tested, and must be regarded as experimental. Long-term use may be associated with significant serious side-effects.

INFECTION: INTERFERON AND INTERFERON INDUCERS

Interferon: Natural Interferon-α or -β; Recombinant Interferon-α or β; Intrathecal Interferon-β

Description: Interferons (IFNs) are substances produced by cells in response to a variety of inducers, including viruses; they are capable of protecting surrounding cells from viral infection. IFN-α is produced by natural killer lymphocytes (NK cells); IFN-β by fibroblast cells; IFN-γ is produced by T-lymphocytes that have been activated by an antigen or virus. Natural IFNs are difficult to produce in large quantities. Most IFNs now used in treatment have been produced in large quantities by "recombinant DNA" techniques.

Rationale: The various types of IFN not only have the ability to protect cells from viral infection, but also have complex effects on immune regulation. The decision to try IFN as therapy in MS was based on the theory that MS may be due to a viral infection, even though there is little evidence to support this notion (see page 11: What Is the Cause of Multiple Sclerosis?). A more recent finding that a large proportion of MS exacerbations are preceded by common viral infections might be another reason to use IFNs. Also, EAE, which may be an animal model for MS, is inhibited by IFN treatment.

Evaluation: Natural IFN-α was used in a controlled study in 24 patients; they received IFN for 6 months, nothing for 6 months, placebo for 6 months, and nothing for another 6 months. There was a weak effect in reducing the number of exacerbations during the IFN treatment period, but progression of MS was not stopped. Another controlled trial of IFN-β given by repeated injection into the spinal fluid for 6 months reported an approximate 60% decrease in exacerbations in the 34 IFN-treated patients in comparison to only about a 25% decrease in 35 placebo-treated patients. The entire study lasted 2 years.

Risks/Costs: Recombinant IFN costs should be lower than that of natural IFN. Side-effects are common and include fever, malaise, nausea, hair loss, depression, and reduction in the white blood cell count.

Conclusion: Further studies are necessary to determine the usefulness of IFN in MS. The effects of IFN-α were encouraging but slight. IFN-β may be effective by injection subcutaneously or intramuscularly, and studies using these simpler routes are in progress.

In the opinion of the Committee, the rationale of this therapy is plausible, but it has not been adequately tested, and must be regarded as experimental. Its use carries significant risk. It is very expensive.

INFECTION: INTERFERON AND INTERFERON INDUCERS

Interferon-γ

Description: This type of IFN is naturally produced by T-lymphocytes that have been activated by exposure to an antigen to which they are sensitive. It is also produced by recombinant DNA technology. This type of IFN not only has antiviral effects, but also the important effect of enhancing antigen recognition. Sensitized T-lymphocytes and macrophages cannot attack their target unless the target cells express histocompatibility antigens (HLA) on their surface membranes. IFN-γ induces the expression of HLA antigens on cell surfaces.

Rationale: The reason for a trial of this type of IFN in MS was the same as for other IFNs, namely, that MS might be related to a viral infection.

Evaluation: In the only trial of IFN-γ in MS, 7 of 18 patients experienced an exacerbation during a 1-month treatment period, a very high rate of worsening.

Conclusion: IFN-γ is not appropriate therapy, because it appears to make MS worse.

In the opinion of the Committee, this therapy should not be used because of reported harmful effects.

INFECTION: INTERFERON AND INTERFERON INDUCERS

Tilorone, Poly-ICLC, Staphage Lysate

Description: These are drugs that stimulate the production of IFN, both α and γ. Poly-ICLC is a synthetic nucleic acid analog. Staphage lysate is produced by dissolving a culture of *Staphylococcus aureus* with bacteriophage (a virus that kills bacteria).

Rationale: The same as for IFN.

Evaluation: Tilorone has been tested in MS with little or no apparent effect. Also, in a study of nine patients with rapidly progressive MS given repeated doses of Poly-ICLC, the disease appeared to be improved in five, and stabilized for a time in three; but two of the latter deteriorated later while still on treatment. In eight patients with slowly progressive MS, disease seemed stabilized in four, but the others withdrew because of unpleasant side-effects.

Risks/Costs: The drugs are less expensive than IFN, but produce toxic side-effects including high fever, nausea, and lassitude.

Conclusion: These drugs should not be used, except possibly in a clinical trial. They induce the production of IFN-γ, which has been shown in one other study to increase the frequency of MS exacerbations.

In the opinion of the Committee, this therapy should not be used because of reported harmful effects.

INFECTION: ANTIVIRAL CHEMOTHERAPY

Methisoprinol (Inosiplex, Isoprinosine)

Description: Methisoprinol is a synthetic immunomodulating and antiviral drug, a complex of inosine and *p*-acetamidobenzoic acid. There is evidence that it is immunostimulating when the immune system is depressed, but not when it is overactive. It has been studied as an antiviral agent for more than two decades.

Rationale: Immune modulation and reputed antiviral properties; the latter might be useful in view of reports that MS attacks are triggered by certain common viral infections.

Evaluation: Only two uncontrolled pilot trials have been reported. Patients were reported to do better during the trial than during the period before it. The authors of the last trial involving 25 patients believe a controlled trial is necessary to prove efficacy.

Risks/Costs: In the largest trial reported, treatment was given intermittently for 2 years, and no significant side effects were reported except occasional slight nausea. Slight rises in serum uric acid may occur. Costs are undetermined.

Conclusion: A controlled clinical trial will be necessary to determine efficacy.

In the opinion of the Committee, the rationale of this therapy is plausible, but the results of controlled trials are not yet available, and it must be regarded as investigational. It is relatively free of serious adverse side-effects during long-term use.

INFECTION: ANTIVIRAL CHEMOTHERAPY

Amantadine (Symmetrel)

Description: Amantadine is a synthetic chemical chiefly useful in prevention of infections by the influenza type A virus. Certain other viruses (influenza C, rubella, and Sendai) are inhibited also; some effect in herpes zoster (shingles) has also been reported. The drug also facilitates release of dopamine from nerve endings in the CNS, and is thus widely used in parkinsonism.

Rationale: There is little evidence that MS is directly caused by infection with any virus. However, some common viral infections precede attacks of MS in about one-third of cases and are considered a risk factor (see page 11: What Is the Cause of Multiple Sclerosis?) Possibly if some of these infections could be prevented, some new plaques of MS could also be prevented.

Evaluation: In an early double-blind trial, amantadine-treated patients fared better than control patients over 40 weeks, but the difference was not statistically significant. In a more recent study reported in 1987, 34 patients completed a 2-year trial: treated patients had significantly fewer relapses than controls, although there was no effect on disability levels during this relatively short study.

Risks/Costs: Amantadine usually produces no side-effects in a dose of 100 mg twice daily, and its safety has been documented in many thousands of patients, especially those with parkinsonism. Rarely, the drug can cause confusion, hallucinations, or urinary retention, especially in the elderly.

Conclusion: Amantadine is a relatively safe drug that deserves further study in the treatment of MS in view of published reports that it can reduce the frequency of exacerbations. Some studies suggest that it may also relieve the sense of overwhelming fatigue common in many MS patients.

In the opinion of the Committee, the rationale of this therapy is plausible, but it has not been adequately tested, and must be regarded as experimental. It is relatively free of serious adverse side-effects during long-term use.

INFECTION: ANTIVIRAL CHEMOTHERAPY

Acyclovir (Zovirax)

Description: Acyclovir is a synthetic drug that can be given intravenously or orally.

Rationale: It is a relatively new drug, proven to be effective in preventing and treating infections with herpes viruses, including herpes simplex (cold sores, type I; genital herpes, type II), varicella-zoster (the virus of chicken pox and shingles), cytamegalovirus, and Epstein-Barr virus (EBV, the virus of infectious mononucleosis). It does not, however, eliminate these viruses, which live in many people in latent form and only occasionally cause illness. Cold sores and shingles are common complications of immunosuppressive drug therapy. No relationship between herpes viruses and MS has been proven, although higher antibody titers occur to varicella-zoster and EBV in MS patients as a group. MS patients have many fewer cold sores than controls, according to one study. A rationale for the use of any antiviral drug in MS is the observation that MS attacks may be precipitated by infection with certain common viruses (see page 11: What Is the Cause of Multiple Sclerosis?).

Evaluation: Two trials are planned, but no results have yet been reported.

Risks/Costs: In general, acyclovir is a relatively safe drug. High doses are reported to interfere with sperm production. The drug should be used with caution in women of childbearing age because there are not good data about the effect on the pregnancy. High doses can cause temporary kidney function impairment because the drug may precipitate in the kidney tubules.

Conclusion: There is no information yet on the possible usefulness of this antiviral drug in MS; the results of planned trials are awaited.

In the opinion of the Committee, the rationale of this therapy is plausible, but it has not been adequately tested, and must be regarded as experimental. It is relatively free of serious adverse side-effects during short-term use. Long-term use may be associated with significant serious side-effects.

V

Symptomatic and General Management of Multiple Sclerosis

This chapter will discuss what can be done to treat some of the symptoms of MS and enhance the quality of life for patients. As yet, there is no general agreement that any treatment exists to cure or retard the progress of the disease; nonetheless, the symptoms and complications can be treated, some more easily than others. The Medical Management Committee of the IFMSS considered a number of areas of management and agreed on certain commonly accepted principles in the symptomatic medical management of MS patients. The areas to be considered include (a) motor disturbances, including spasticity, weakness, and ataxia; (b) pain; (c) fatigue; (d) bladder, bowel, and sexual disturbances; (e) cognitive and psychological symptoms; (f) vaccinations; (g) diet; (h) the treatment of certain paroxysmal symptoms; and (i) the ideal: comprehensive MS care centers.

MOTOR DISTURBANCES

Spasticity

Spasticity is an *increase in muscle tone,* common to many neurological diseases, but especially frequent in MS. There are two

---

Material for this chapter was contributed by the Medical Management Committee, Dr. Donald W. Paty, Chairman.

manifestations of spasticity that require treatment. The first is *phasic spasms:* these can be either flexor or extensor; they occur most commonly in the legs, especially at night. Such spasms are very detrimental to the balance of the patient and can also be very painful. The second form of spasticity is the *sustained increase in tone* that interferes with walking in ambulatory patients, and interferes with hygiene and nursing care in bedridden patients.

In evaluating spasticity it is important to assess the patient's function, not just the neurological examination. There are instances, for example, when spasticity is actually beneficial to function, as when it aids in the support of weak legs. Overtreatment of spasticity in such a case would be inadvisable. *A physical therapist* can, by the application of cold or by slow stretching exercises, reduce spasticity temporarily, but this usually does not have a sustained effect on the spasticity itself. It does help prevent contractures, however. A contracture is an irreversible shortening of weak, paralyzed, or unused muscles that produces immobility of joints and prevents function, even if the neurological state later improves.

Oral drug therapy can be helpful in the management of spasticity when used carefully. Diazepam, baclofen, and tizanidine are the most useful drugs. One must be careful not to overdose the patient. Overdose in this setting usually means increasing the dose to such a level that weakness becomes a problem. Diazepam has an attendant risk of drug dependence. Dantrolene is another antispastic drug that works by weakening muscles. Because of this and some instances of liver damage, this drug is usually not useful in MS.

Diazepam and baclofen are especially useful for phasic spasms. When these flexor or extensor spasms are worse at night, diazepam is particularly helpful because it not only reduces the frequency of the spasms but also helps maintain sleep. Baclofen and tizanidine are generally the best drugs for spasticity associated with walking; judicious slow increase in the dose can result in significant decrease in the stiffness that interferes with walking. Corticosteroids can also be effective in reducing spasticity, but these drugs are not suitable for long-term use because of complications associated with such therapy. However, short-term use of corticosteroids such as prednisone can be very helpful in reducing spasticity while other measures are being started.

In severe cases, *various surgical destructive procedures* are sometimes used. These include the injection of phenol into the lower spinal canal, into certain peripheral nerves or into the motor endplates of affected muscles: The improvement seen is temporary and treatment may have to be repeated later. The cutting of nerves (neurectomies), nerve roots (rhizotomies), or of the spinal cord itself (myelotomy) has occasionally been used, but these procedures produce permanent deficits in either sensation, bladder function, or strength, and should not be used if there is any possibility of natural improvement. One of the more common and useful surgical procedures is an obturator nerve block or neurectomy, which reduces spasticity when it prevents separation of the thighs for proper nursing care.

Current research includes the trial of very small amounts of intrathecal morphine, administered by an implantable pump, to relieve severe spasticity; more information is necessary before this procedure can be recommended for general use, however.

Weakness and Ataxia (Incoordination)

There is no good treatment for either of these symptoms. However, physical therapists can assist patients to find the most efficient and safe way to use the function that remains. Canes, crutches, and walkers provide various degrees of safety and support. Plastic foot drop braces, molded to fit the foot and calf, worn in the shoe, are among the most useful devices, often improving the gait of patients with moderate degrees of weakness of the feet. Long-leg braces are seldom helpful because of their weight and awkwardness. A wheelchair sometimes becomes necessary for long trips, years before it is necessary for ordinary everyday activities. For patients with serious weakness or ataxia, motorized wheelchairs provide a considerable degree of independence. *Occupational therapists* can help some patients who have a loss of manual dexterity adapt to their condition by the use of special tools and devices.

The severe tremor of the arms or head that occurs in some patients is not easily treated. Some have advocated isonicotinic acid hydrazide (INH) in large doses, or clonazepam (Clonopin). A vitamin B ^{6} (pyridoxine) supplement must be used with INH, and clonazepam is a very sedative drug for many patients. A trial of these agents may be warranted in some patients, but the success rate is low. Surgical procedures on the brain, such as thalamotomy, have been used successfully in some patients, but such procedures are fraught with the risk of increasing mental impairment or difficulty in swallowing.

PAIN

Patients with MS commonly complain of pain but this symptom has largely been neglected. Three kinds of pain can be identified: (a) *musculoskeletal pain:* this is often related to musculoskeletal imbalance. Moderately disabled patients may have back pain due to incorrect posture and poorly designed wheelchairs. Pain due to osteoporosis, compression fractures of vertebrae, arthritis in the hips and neck, contractures, and spasticity are all considered in this category; (b) *paroxysmal pain:* the classical example is the sharp stabbing face pain of trigeminal neuralgia (tic douloureux), but other paroxysmal pains can occur, often in the general distribution of a nerve root; (c) *chronic neurogenic pain:* these pains are often described as constant boring, burning, constricting, or intense tingling that are present in a diffuse distribution, especially in the legs.

The treatment of *musculoskeletal pain* is to correct the causative problem, if possible. When this is not possible such pains may respond to aspirin (which has been shown to be safe in MS), or acetaminophen. The newer NSAIDs should be used only under the direction of a physician (see page 32), with the understanding that they have not had extensive study in MS patients, and that there are theoretical reasons to suspect, and at least one report, that some may worsen MS. The treatment of *paroxysmal pains* such as trigeminal neuralgia is usually with carbamazepine or other anticonvulsant drugs; specific surgical approaches also exist if these drugs are ineffective.

The treatment of *chronic neurogenic pain* (presumably arising because of the location of certain plaques in the spinal cord or brain) is difficult; such pain tends to be persistent and respond poorly. The tricyclic antidepressant drugs, e.g., amitriptyline, or the monoamine oxidase (MAO) inhibitor class of antidepressant drugs can be helpful in some cases. Physical methods of treatment such as peripheral nerve stimulation (see page 161: Transcutaneous Nerve Stimulation) may also be effective in some patients. Narcotic analgesics should be avoided, if possible, because of the risk of addiction in treating such chronic pain; these drugs also worsen constipation. However, sometimes combinations of codeine with either aspirin or acetaminophen must be used for long periods because of the intensity of certain chronic pains; such management should avoid increases in the dose of codeine and may be the only practical means available for pain control.

FATIGUE

Two types of fatigue can be distinguished. A *persistent sense of tiredness* may prevent the accomplishment of even light tasks. In the other form the patient will generally feel well at rest, but will be overcome by a generalized sensation of fatigue, usually after a few minutes of physical activity; this is termed *fatigability,* and it will often disappear after a short rest. The most common form of fatigability is in the legs, when the strength in the legs will deteriorate after walking for a short distance. Some patients overexert or try to exceed the limits of their ability by walking with canes when they should be using a motorized wheelchair for long distances. Fatigability may affect the sensory system also; for example, with prolonged reading, visual ability and clarity deteriorate, but return after a short rest.

Both types of fatigue are common in MS, and both are thought to have both physiological and psychological components. The physiological aspects of fatigue, especially the phenomenon of fatigability, may be related to a marginal ability to conduct nerve impulses through plaques, and should be distinguished from psychological fatigue. The latter is characterized by listlessness, languor, apathy, and depression, and may respond well to antidepressant drugs. Fatigue and other symptoms in MS are made worse characteristically by a hot bath, increased body temperature, and hot weather. Sometimes fatigue may be the most important aspect of disabilty in MS and interferes considerably with activities of daily living.

The most important approach to treatment of fatigue is to *teach patients to pace themselves properly.* They must not take on excessive physical activity without the ability to rest. Another approach is to *avoid even small increases in body temperature* by avoiding long periods of vigorous exercise and warm surroundings. Repeated cold baths or showers may help. Air conditioning is important in hot climates.

Several *drugs* have been reported to help in some, but not all, patients. These include amantadine; about half of patients taking this drug believe it helps maintain energy. Pemoline (Cylert) has been reported to be beneficial in about two-thirds of patients. Antidepressant drugs can be helpful in some cases. A recent trial with 4-aminopyridine suggested that this compound can reduce fatigue and improve strength and balance for a few minutes or hours; it is still under investigation, and is not generally available.

BLADDER, BOWEL, AND SEXUAL DISTURBANCES

Bladder Disturbances

There are at least three distinct kinds of bladder function disturbance in MS: (a) *a failure to store urine;* the bladder wall becomes irritable, the bladder is small and tends to empty itself frequently. The symptoms are urgency, frequency, and incontinence; (b) *failure to empty urine:* the bladder is large, as is the volume of urine retained in the bladder, and there is poor emptying: infection is especially common; (c) *a combination of (a) and (b):* this occurs when there is an incoordination between the muscles attempting to empty the bladder and the sphincter muscles that try to store urine: here again, the postvoiding residual urine volume tends to be high, and infection is common.

The initial symptoms of urinary disturbance in MS can be frequency, urgency, incontinence, hesitancy, and (rarely) retention. Urinary frequency may occur even when the bladder is large and retains large volumes, as an overflow phenomenon. Some of these symptoms can often respond very dramatically to drugs, but one must be careful not to make the condition worse by increasing the tendency to pool urine in a large, weak bladder.

Suggested approaches to urinary symptoms are to (a) *monitor carefully for infection;* this means periodic urinalysis even in patients without urinary symptoms. When infection occurs, antibiotics should be used for a period and then discontinued; long-term antibiotic treatment is usually not useful. A urinary antiseptic such as methenamine mandelate or huppurate (Mandelamine, Hiprex, Urex) can be used for long periods and works by producing formaldehyde in acid urine. Acidification of the urine helps prevent infection, and is especially important in patients taking methenamine; it can be accomplished by the chronic use of vitamin C or cranberry juice; citrus juices should be avoided; (b) *know the residual urine volume;* excessive post-voiding residual urine in the bladder is detrimental and tends to promote infection, although volumes less than 100 ml are often well tolerated; the residual urine after voiding can be determined directly by catheterization, by an ultrasound device, or by intravenous pyelography (special radiography of the kidneys and bladder).

When urinary frequency is the main problem and there is a low residual urine volume, a trial of therapy with an agent capable of reducing the irritability of the bladder wall is warranted. Suitable drugs for this purpose are propantheline (Pro-Banthine), dicyclomine (Bentyl), oxybutynin (Ditropan), imipramine (Tofranil), or isopropamide (Darbid).

When there is a high postvoiding residual urine volume, intermittent clean catheterization is necessary several times each day. If the patient can do the catheterization it is preferable; but if the patient is disabled by poor coordination or strength in the hands, catheterization by a caregiver can substitute.

Sometimes, in the third type of bladder disturbance mentioned above, in which there is incoordination between the bladder wall and the sphincter, a drug capable of reducing bladder wall irritability (see above) may be combined with intermittent clean catheterization. Constant drainage by the use of an indwelling catheter is to be avoided because it always leads to infection or other complications. Adult diapers are preferable to constant catheter drainage. In males, condom catheters can be very useful both at night, and during periods away from home, to avoid incontinence.

Bowel Problems

Constipation is very common in disabled patients, and is made worse by a reluctance to drink enough water because of associated urinary frequency or incontinence. Constipation can usually be prevented by adequate fluid intake, and a high-fiber intake, as produced by ingesting bran cereals; some patients prefer more refined high-fiber products such as methylcellulose (Cologel) or psyllium hydrophilic colloid (Metamucil, Perdiem Plain).

Fecal incontinence is much less frequent, and usually a temporary symptom, occurring primarily with diarrhea as a result of other illness, laxative overdose, or dietary causes. Treatment is the same as for diarrhea.

Sexual Dysfunction

Sexual dysfunction is common in MS patients. When it occurs, it does so primarily in those who also have bladder dysfunction. In the absence of the latter, psychological causes should be considered.

In the male, failure of erection is the main problem; often the symptom is intermittent. If permanent, various types of penile implants may be considered. Recently, however, it has been shown that injection of small amounts of papaverine into the penis with a fine needle can produce satisfactory erections; this should be attempted only with the detailed instructions of a physician, usually a urologist. Electrostimulation of ejaculation may allow neurologically impaired men to father children. In women, anorgasmy is the most common complaint; apparently this symptom may occasionally be helped by the use of electric vibrating devices.

Urological and psychological counseling is an important aspect of the management of serious sexual dysfunction.

PSYCHOLOGICAL AND COGNITIVE DISTURBANCES

These functions can be impaired as MS advances; rarely, MS can present with depression, mania, or a cognitive disturbance such as memory loss and/or dementia. The effectiveness of a medical and physical rehabilitation program in a specific patient may be diminished by the presence of severe cognitive or psychiatric abnormalities, but in these cases cognitive/psychiatric rehabilitation may be attempted. Formal neuropsychological testing may be helpful in arriving at the proper diagnosis.

When depression complicates MS, there is often a seeming exaggeration of the neurological disability beyond objective signs. When depression is a major feature, standard antidepressant therapy is often effective, using either tricyclic antidepressants or MAO inhibitors. When there is underlying cognitive abnormality, antidepressant treatment is much less effective, but it should still be attempted.

The family and the various caregivers should be made aware of what underlying disturbance is present. Sometimes when psychological or cognitive problems are present, the family may misinterpret, and feel that the patient is willfully resisting their help. When caregivers are given specific knowledge of the underlying problem, they can be much more understanding and supportive.

Early in the course of MS patients are often needlessly referred for psychiatric care with an erroneous diagnosis of hysteria, because symptoms are not associated with objective changes on neurological examination. Later, when the diagnosis of MS is well established, physicians and others again may consider the symptoms exaggerated for psychological reasons;

sometimes this is true, especially when MS is complicated by depression. In other instances, however, a patient's perception of disordered nervous system function may simply be more acute than the physician's ability to detect new lesions.

VACCINATIONS

MS is thought to be an autoimmune disease. Therefore, vaccinations and other immune manipulations could be considered potentially harmful. Epidemiological studies have not shown that vaccinations can reproducibly precipitate worsening in MS, but it is generally thought that the theoretical implication of vaccinations is enough to recommend caution. Two recent studies of influenza vaccination showed that this vaccine can probably be administered with relative safety, but more extensive studies will have to be done.

For the individual patient, the recommendations would be to *follow local medical advice*. It is probably better to avoid vaccination unless there is a specific reason not to do so. Typhoid vaccine, for example, will increase the general population level of resistance to typhoid infection, but the protection for the individual is very much less than for the population. Vaccines such as typhoid, then, would best be avoided, unless one is to travel in an especially high-risk zone for the disease. Influenza and pneumonia vaccines, however, are probably quite effective in reducing the chance of these diseases in disabled patients, and should be considered if the physician feels that there is a high risk from these illnesses.

DIET

Recommendations as to diet abound in the lay literature on MS. Suffice it to say that no diet has been proven to be beneficial to the disease process, with the possible exception of a diet high in PUFA, which have shown a marginal effect in some studies.

Excessive calories should be avoided. The most commonly followed diet is one that is low in animal fats and dairy products. This diet is generally very healthful because of the implications of fatty acids for the cardiovascular system. So long as adequate nutrition is maintained, one cannot argue against a low-fat approach to dietary management.

PAROXYSMAL SYMPTOMS

A small number of patients with MS develop one or more paroxysmal symptoms. Paroxysmal pain in the face has been considered above, and occurs in approximately 5% of patients. Epileptic seizures occur in approximately 2% of patients. Other phenomena such as painful tonic spasms, paroxysmal weakness, paroxysmal loss of sensation, and paroxysmal dysarthria (slurred speech) and ataxia occur much less frequently.

In all cases the symptoms come on suddenly, last only a few seconds to a minute, and disappear quickly. They may recur several times each day. All such symptoms usually respond promptly to anticonvulsants such as carbamazepine or phenytoin in the same doses used to control convulsive seizures. Such paroxysmal symptoms, with the exception of convulsive seizures themselves, are usually self limited, often lasting a few weeks and then subsiding; thus, they seldom require prolonged therapy.

COMPREHENSIVE LONG-TERM MANAGEMENT AND REHABILITATION

A comprehensive MS center providing accurate information, treatment, and advice to patients and their families is an ideal. An intensive, short-term, multidisciplinary rehabilitation approach can yield considerable functional improvement even in patients with severe handicaps. This beneficial effect can then be maintained on an outpatient basis.

In moderately disabled patients, exercise programs tailored to their individual needs can be very beneficial, recognizing that the fatigue limit of that individual must not be exceeded. One cannot define an "ideal" regimen of physiotherapy for MS patients because of the fluctuating nature of the disease and the low tolerance of many patients for exercise.

There is no doubt that long-term management of MS is quite different from the management of other chronic neurological diseases, and is best done as a multidisciplinary approach to the problem in a specialized unit. The management of more severely disabled patients is more difficult when such units do not exist. The ultimate goal should be to keep the patient at home with the family as much as possible, but intermittent admission into a specialized inpatient service can be beneficial to both patients and their families. It is important to be direct, truthful, and supportive in long-term management. Denial, although an effective psychological protection in certain difficult short-term medical situations, does not work very well in chronic disabling disorders such as MS.

SYMPTOMATIC TREATMENTS AFFECTING SPASTICITY

Baclofen (Lioresal)

Description: Baclofen is an oral drug, available by prescription.

Rationale: In many patients with spasticity, the stiffness of the legs as well as the slowness and restricted range of movement are an important part of the interference with walking. Such patients may benefit from reduction in spasticity. Baclofen appears to act on certain nerve receptors in the spinal cord, thereby reducing the excessive reflex activity that underlies spasticity.

Evaluation: Baclofen, diazepam, tizanidine, and dantrolene are effective in reducing spasticity. Baclofen and tizanidine do this by action on the spinal cord, whereas the site of action of dantrolene is in the muscle.

Overall, baclofen is considered the most effective agent for spasticity. It may improve bladder and bowel control as well. The dose may have to exceed recommendations in about one-third of patients to achieve benefits.

Risks/Costs: These are similar to those for diazepam and tizanidine. Baclofen may produce transient drowsiness, but usually less than diazepam. Abrupt withdrawal of the drug after prolonged use may be followed by seizures or a period of hallucinations.

Conclusion: Baclofen is the most effective and least toxic drug available for reducing spasticity in patients with MS.

In the opinion of the Committee, the efficacy of this therapy in selected patients has been demonstrated. It is relatively free of serious adverse side-effects during long-term use.

SYMPTOMATIC TREATMENTS AFFECTING SPASTICITY

Diazepam (Valium)

Description: Diazepam is an oral drug, available by prescription.

Rationale: Similar to that for baclofen. Diazepam reduces spasticity by action on the CNS.

Evaluation: Diazepam, and dantrolene and baclofen as well, are effective in reducing spasticity. The margin between reduction of spasticity and increasing weakness is small, and varies from time to time. Individual patients vary in their relative response to the three drugs. Overall, baclofen is considered the most effective. The tranquilizing and sedative effects of diazepam may be of value in their own right in depressed or anxious patients.

Risks/Costs: Similar to dantrolene. Valium, in doses large enough to affect spasticity, often has a sedative effect, and may produce drowsiness or dizziness. Prolonged use promotes drug dependency.

Conclusion: This drug is effective in reducing spasticity in MS.

In the opinion of the Committee, the efficacy of this therapy in selected patients has been demonstrated. Long-term use may be associated with significant serious side-effects.

SYMPTOMATIC TREATMENTS AFFECTING SPASTICITY

Tizanidine (Sirdalut)

Description: An oral drug, widely used in Europe.

Rationale: Similar to that for baclofen. Tizanidine reduces muscle tone by an action at the level of the spinal cord, but has little effect on reflex spasm.

Evaluation: There have been a number of studies establishing the efficacy of tizanidine, especially for muscle stiffness and "clonus." It is sometimes effective in reducing spasticity in patients refractory to other agents. Conjoint use with low doses of baclofen is said to produce an optimal effect with fewer side effects.

Risks/Costs: Minor. Tizanidine is less sedative than diazepam or baclofen.

Conclusion: Tizanidine is useful in the treatment of spasticity.

In the opinion of the Committee, the efficacy of this therapy in selected patients has been demonstrated. It is relatively free of serious adverse side-effects during long-term use.

SYMPTOMATIC TREATMENTS AFFECTING SPASTICITY

Dantrolene Sodium (Dantrium)

Description: An oral drug available by prescription.

Rationale: Similar to baclofen. Dantrolene appears to reduce spasticity by interfering with the excitation of muscle fibers to contract, thus producing in essence some weakness. A trial of the drug is usually necessary to determine whether a particular patient obtains benefit.

Evaluation: Dantrolene, and diazepam and baclofen as well, are effective in reducing spasticity. The margin between reduction of spasticity and increasing weakness is small and varies from time to time. Individual patients vary in their relative response to the individual drugs. Overall, baclofen is considered the most effective, with diazepam being second best.

Risks/Costs: In some patients, spasticity may help compensate for ataxia of gait or weakness of the legs. Reducing spasticity in such a case may result in worsening of ability to walk. The most serious risk in use of dantrolene is the possible development of liver damage. Also, long-term use may produce pleural effusion (fluid in the chest).

Conclusion: Dantrolene is effective in reducing spasticity, but carries a threat of liver damage and pleural effusions.

In the opinion of the Committee, this therapy has been demonstrated to have limited usefulness in selected patients. Its use carries significant risk.

SYMPTOMATIC TREATMENTS AFFECTING SPASTICITY

Ketazolam (Unakalm, Anxon)

Description: A drug similar to diazepam (Valium).

Rationale: As for diazepam. Ketazolam is said to produce fewer side-effects.

Evaluation: In a double-blind, crossover study, ketazolam was shown to be as effective as diazepam in relieving spasticity and was significantly better than a placebo. It was believed by the authors to offer a safe and clinically useful alternative in the treatment of spasticity.

Risks/Costs: Unknown.

Conclusion: The evidence presented suggests that ketazolam may be useful in the treatment of spasticity.

In the opinion of the Committee, this therapy has been demonstrated to have limited usefulness in selected patients. Long-term use may be associated with significant serious side-effects.

SYMPTOMATIC TREATMENTS AFFECTING SPASTICITY

Progabide

Description: An oral drug, not available in the United States.

Rationale: Progabide acts in the CNS on nerve cells with receptors for gamma-aminobutyric acid, a well-known inhibitory neurotransmitter. It is an effective antispastic drug.

Evaluation: A Danish pilot study (double-blind, crossover) on 14 MS patients showed a beneficial therapeutic effect on spasticity during a 2-week period of treatment. An American pilot study also showed significant objective decrease in spasticity in treated patients relative to controls. However, in studies carried out in France it was found to be less effective than baclofen.

Risks/Costs: Progabide leads to liver damage in a significant proportion of patients and even to occasional fatalities from hepatitis.

Conclusion: This drug should not be used.

In the opinion of the Committee, this therapy should not be used because of reported harmful effects.

SYMPTOMATIC TREATMENTS AFFECTING SPASTICITY

Thyrotropin-Releasing Hormone

Description: A peptide hormone, injected daily by the subcutaneous route.

Rationale: A new alternative drug useful for spasticity and lacking the side-effects associated with commonly used anti-spasticity agents. The mechanism of action of thyrotropin-releasing hormone (TRH) is uncertain but appears to involve lowering the level of excitability of those spinal cord nerve cells (lower motor neuron) that innervate muscle and control movement.

Evaluation: In a double-blind, crossover study, ketazolam was shown to cause slight to marked improvement of spasticity, muscle cramps, and spasms in a number of diseases including MS. In "pure" spasticity, not associated with damage of the lower motor neuron, TRH also lessens fatigability and weakness. An effect is seen within 1 to 2 h of drug administration and lasts several days. More extensive trials are in progress, as well as attempts to identify TRH derivatives or analogs with superior therapeutic potential or a longer-lasting effect.

Risks/Costs: Cost is moderate. TRH produces no significant side-effects. At very high dose, it gives a transient "autorefractory state," in which responsiveness to the drug is lost.

Conclusion: A judgment as to the potential usefulness of TRH in MS awaits the publications of further trials.

In the opinion of the Committee, there appears to be no generally accepted scientific basis for use of this therapy. It has never been tested in a proper controlled trial. It is relatively free of serious adverse side-effects during short-term use.

SYMPTOMATIC TREATMENTS AFFECTING SPASTICITY

Cannabis (Marijuana, Hashish, Tetrahydrocannabinol)

Description: A group of natural substances extracted from leaves or flowers of *Cannibis sativa* var. *indica* and related plants.

Rationale: A number of patients with MS reported that smoking marijuana improved their spasticity. This agent also affects the smoker's emotional state.

Evaluation: Tetrahydrocannabinol (THC), an active ingredient in marijuana, and placebos were used in a small double-blind controlled study of spasticity. The spasticity scores in seven of nine patients on the active drug were found to be lower than for those on placebo. Two patients reported a "high" while on THC and one reported a "high" while on placebo, showing that the doses of drug used were not psychoactive. In another study, two of eight severely disabled patients showed improved coordination and reduced tremor. A current double-blind trial is testing the effect of marijuana on posture, gait, and neurological status in a larger series of patients.

Risks/Costs: No significant side-effects were reported in the limited trials. No serious long-term effects have been proven to result from use of this drug. However, clinical experience suggests that long-term heavy pot smoking may impair memory and be associated with personality changes. It would appear that other drugs may reduce spasticity with fewer side-effects than marijuana. Marijuana and its active ingredients have not been approved for use in treatment of spasticity.

Conclusion: Further studies are required to determine whether marijuana has a clinically useful effect on MS. In view of the possible toxic effects of long-term use, its use cannot be recommended.

In the opinion of the Committee, there appears to be no generally accepted scientific basis for use of this therapy. It has never been tested in a proper controlled trial. Long-term use may be associated with significant serious side-effects.

SYMPTOMATIC TREATMENTS AFFECTING SPASTICITY

Surgical Manipulations

Description: Phenol or alcohol injections into nerves, cutting of nerves (neurotomy), or nerve roots (rhizotomy), or cutting of the spinal cord (myelotomy).

Rationale: In a few patients, spasticity is severe and does not respond to medical treatment. Such patients, or patients with total bladder and bowel dysfunction, may be considered for surgical procedures.

Evaluation: Injection of individual nerves with phenol produces a selective block of these nerves and weakness of the muscles they supply. The effect of the injection may wear off after about 6 months. Occasionally, for more widespread effect, phenol injection of nerves intraspinally has been done. Cutting a nerve or nerve roots may modify extreme spasticity. Cutting of muscles or tendons and transplanting of tendons may also be considered. On rare occasions, a lengthwise cutting of the spinal cord is performed to interrupt the reflex circuit that sustains spasticity. Before such destructive operative procedures are considered,the spasticity should be extreme and should have been present long enough to be certain that a remission will not occur, ordinarily at least 2 years.

Risks/Costs: Surgical procedures are effective at the cost of increased weakness. They are expensive as well. Phenol injections may occasionally provoke thrombophlebitis (clotting in nearby veins).

Conclusion: Surgical procedures may help MS patients with severe spasticity that does not respond to medical treatment.

In the opinion of the Committee, the efficacy of this therapy in selected patients has been demonstrated. Its use carries significant risk. It is very expensive.

SYMPTOMATIC TREATMENTS AFFECTING CONDUCTION

Cold

Description: Cooling, as by immersion in a swimming pool.

Rationale: Exposure to heat, as in hot weather or a hot bath, produces dramatic temporary worsening of neurologic symptoms in many MS patients, whereas cooling tends to have the opposite effect. Experimentally, borderline conducting nerve fibers are blocked with small temperature increases, whereas some blocked fibers will conduct when the temperature is decreased.

Evaluation: Some patients are able to increase their ability to function by general body cooling in a swimming pool, but this is a temporary effect. Patients should prevent temporary worsening by avoiding heat. Rarely, excessive heat exposure has apparently led to permanent worsening.

Risks/Costs: Negligible.

Conclusion: Judicious use of cold is an adjunct to patient management.

In the opinion of the Committee, the efficacy of this therapy in selected patients has been demonstrated. It is relatively free of serious adverse side-effects during long-term use.

SYMPTOMATIC TREATMENTS AFFECTING CONDUCTION

4-Aminopyridine, Tetraethylammonium Chloride, Gallamine Triethiodide (Flaxedil)

Description: Simple chemicals known to bind to potassium ion channel proteins.

Rationale: In physiological experiments with demyelinated nerve, these compounds block potassium movement and prolong the action potential. They thus restore conduction in nerve fibers lacking myelin.

Evaluation: 4-Aminopyridine has been used clinically in the treatment of myasthenia gravis and botulism. It was first tried experimentally in MS in a very small group of patients, but the trial was stopped when seizures were produced. A pilot study has now been completed, with use of lower doses, in 32 patients. There was transient but definite improvement in vision (decreased blind spots, nystagmus), coordination, and strength. These mainly were seen in temperature-sensitive patients, who make up 60% of the MS population. Seizures were not seen at the doses used. There were similar results in another small, uncontrolled study.

For additional discussion of TEA, see page 20: Rationale and Summary of Treatments, Old and Recent: Circulatory Insufficiency. Gallamine triethiodide, a muscle relaxant, has not been tested in MS.

Risks/Costs: Hyperactivity of the nervous system, expressed as convulsions.

Conclusion: This treatment is of interest but remains experimental at the present time.

In the opinion of the Committee, the rationale of this therapy is plausible, but the results of controlled trials are not yet available, and it must be regarded as investigational. Its use carries significant risk.

SYMPTOMATIC TREATMENTS AFFECTING CONDUCTION

Verapamil, Nifedipine, Diltiazem

Description: Drugs in common use for certain forms of heart disease and high blood pressure, available in forms taken by mouth or by injection intravenously.

Rationale: These drugs antagonize movement of calcium ions through specific calcium channels into the cell. They may thus affect nerve cell function, conduction in demyelinated nerve fibers, and the function of the synapse. These drugs are also vasodilators.

Evaluation: Verapamil was injected intravenously in eight MS patients with abnormal visual or brainstem evoked potentials. It produced electrophysiologic improvement without any improvement in clinical state.

Risks/Costs: Costs are moderate.

Conclusion: These drugs are of possible interest, but are unproven at the present time.

In the opinion of the Committee, there appears to be no generally accepted scientific basis for use of this therapy. It has never been tested in a proper controlled trial. It is relatively free of serious adverse side-effects during long-term use.

SYMPTOMATIC TREATMENTS AFFECTING FATIGUE

Amantadine (Symmetrel)

Description: This drug has already been described (see page 88: Infection: Antiviral Chemotherapy). It is a synthetic chemical originally introduced to prevent and treat infections with the influenza A virus. Later it was shown to improve the symptoms of parkinsonism, probably by promoting the release of a neurotransmitter (dopamine) from nerve terminals. In the treatment of parkinsonism it has been used daily in the treatment of thousands of patients for many years, usually without any significant side-effects.

Rationale: Reports have appeared in the medical literature that some patients taking this drug find that it relieves a feeling of chronic fatigue. Some have found this in as many as half of patients.

Evaluation: There are no large-scale controlled studies to substantiate the relief of fatigue, but several small studies have reported this effect.

Risks/Costs: Amantadine usually produces no side-effects in a dose of 100 mg twice daily. Rarely, however, the drug may cause confusion, especially in the elderly, or urinary retention.

Conclusion: Amantadine is a relatively safe drug that seems to alleviate the fatigue of some, but by no means all, MS patients.

In the opinion of the Committee, this therapy has been demonstrated to have limited usefulness in selected patients. It is relatively free of serious adverse side-effects during long-term use.

SYMPTOMATIC TREATMENTS AFFECTING FATIGUE

Pemoline (Cylert)

Description: A synthetic organic chemical that acts as a cerebral stimulant but is structurally dissimilar to dextroamphetamine and methylphenidate and has few or none of their undesirable side effects.

Rationale: Pemoline was developed as a cerebral stimulant and has been used for attention deficit disorder in children and narcolepsy in adults, with good results. On this rationale it has been tried successfully to treat the fatigue of MS.

Evaluation: As yet no double-blind randomized control studies have been reported, but personal communication with some clinicians who have used this report that it is more effective than amantadine and more than 60% of the patients showed moderate or good benefit. There was no report of physiological or psychological dependence, palpatation, or anorexia. Only when the therapeutic range was exceeded did patients report insomnia, which was reversed when the dosage was reduced. Clinical improvement is delayed by 3 to 4 weeks, and the range is usually 18.75 to 187.5 mg given in the morning as a single dose.

Risks/Costs: Toxic side-effects include nervousness, insomnia, and anxiety. The cost is modest.

Conclusion: Pemoline appears to be of value in the treatment of fatigue in some patients with MS.

In the opinion of the Committee, this therapy has been demonstrated to have limited usefulness in selected patients. It is relatively free of serious adverse side-effects during long-term use.

GENERAL MANAGEMENT: DIET

Polyunsaturated Fatty Acids

Description: Dietary supplementation with linolenic acid, linoleic acid, sunflower seed oil, safflower seed oil, or evening primrose oil (Naudicelle) (Gamma Prim).

Rationale: Linolenic and linoleic acids are essential PUFAs that can be used by the body to synthesize other fatty acids and are elements of myelin in the CNS. Some studies have reported low levels of linoleic acid in the serum of MS patients, whereas other studies have shown normal levels. It has also been suggested that PUFA may exert some immunosuppressive effect, because large doses of PUFA protect guinea pigs against experimental autoimmune encephalomyelitis, regarded as a model for MS.

Evaluation: Preliminary studies with PUFA suggested a possible favorable therapeutic effect. There have been three recent scientifically controlled, sizable studies of the use of PUFA in MS. The treatment was followed for at least 2 years in each case. Various sources of PUFA were used, including sunflower seed oil, evening primrose oil (Naudicelle), and safflower seed oil. One study reported some reduction in frequency of exacerbations. Another study reported some reduction in the severity and duration of individual attacks, but no change in their frequency. The third study failed to find any favorable effect. However, a recent reanalysis of the data from the three trials led to the conclusion that treated patients with minimal disability (at the time of entry into trial) had less increase in disability than controls. In addition, treatment reduced the severity and duration of relapses at all levels of disability and duration of illness (at entry into trial).

In one clinic, large doses of PUFA, in the form of Naudicelle, were supplemented by colchicine administered orally twice a day on the ground that it might affect prostaglandin production and possibly rates of calcium entry in stimulated immune cells. In a pilot study lasting 6 months, four of six chronic stable patients were reported to show improvement on the regimen, whereas three of eight given PUFA only showed a slight improvement.

Risks/Costs: No significant toxic effects have been reported. According to our experience, some patients find pure oil distasteful and may better tolerate emulsions, spreads, or capsules. Some patients develop diarrhea. Long-term effects of high PUFA intake are unknown. The cost of dietary supplementation with linoleic acid is modest. Studies have shown, however, that colchicine has prominent side-effects and the safety of its long-term use is questionable.

Conclusion: On the basis of studies conducted to date, dietary supplementation with linoleic acid or with natural oils containing PUFA appears to slow progression and reduce the severity and duration of MS exacerbations without affecting their frequency. The effect is apparently a very modest one, because it has been difficult to demonstrate in some studies.

In the opinion of the Committee, this therapy may have some efficacy, but the evidence is conflicting, and it must be regarded as investigational. It is relatively free of serious adverse side-effects during long-term use.

GENERAL MANAGEMENT: DIET

Fatty Acids of Fish Oil

Description: Dietary supplementation with eicosapentaenoic (timnodonic) acid and docosahexaenoic (clupanodonic) acid in fish oils.

Rationale: Eskimos consume large amounts of fish and other marine animals, in whose flesh these unusual PUFAs are present at high concentration. This population does not get MS and shows decreased levels of ischemic heart disease. Experimental observations have established that consumption of fish oil PUFA markedly inhibits some of the key elements in inflammation, notably the production and action of prostaglandins, thomboxane, and leukotrienes.

Evaluation: A large multicenter controlled, double-blind trial of the effect of dietary supplementation with PUFA in Great Britain made use of fish oil, and has been completed. There was a trend in favor of the treatment that did not, however, reach accepted levels of statistical significance ($p = 0.07$).

Risks/Costs: Many patients find the fishy taste, associated with large doses of the oil (even when taken in capsules), unpleasant. Costs are modest.

Conclusion: The evidence suggests that fish oil may be of some benefit, although the data is not conclusive. As with other PUFAs the effect is apparently very modest.

In the opinion of the Committee, this therapy may have some efficacy, but the evidence is conflicting, and it must be regarded as investigational. It is relatively free of serious adverse side-effects during long-term use.

GENERAL MANAGEMENT: DIET

Low-Fat Diet

Description: Regular use of a diet in which animal fats are included at a fixed low level, and vegetable oils at low, intermediate, or high level.

Rationale: Swank pointed out in 1950 that MS is generally more common in populations of the world that have high fat intake. He suggested that high fat ingestion might play a role in the production of MS lesions by causing "sludging" in blood flowing through the CNS.

Evaluation: A large series of MS patients was followed for an average of 17 years on a diet low in animal fat, but supplemented by a moderate amount of vegetable oil. A less rapid progression and a lower death rate were reported, compared with the natural course of MS described in neurological literature, as well as reduction in the frequency of exacerbations. However, the natural course of MS is usually characterized by more exacerbations early rather than late in the disease. Furthermore, in the study reported, no matched control group was studied concurrently. Most physicians believe that there is little basis for the original hypothesis. White South Africans have a diet very high in saturated animal fats, yet have a low incidence of MS.

Risks/Costs: The low-fat diet is not associated with significant risks.

Conclusion: The low-fat diet has not been proven to be effective in the treatment of MS. It is clear that the diet does not prevent exacerbations or progression. The possibility of a partial or incomplete effect has not been excluded.

In the opinion of the Committee, there appears to be no generally accepted scientific basis for use of this therapy. It has never been tested in a proper controlled trial. It is relatively free of serious adverse side-effects during long-term use.

VI

Miscellaneous and Empirical Treatments

OVERVIEW

History notes that effective treatments for certain diseases have been discovered by accident (e.g., penicillin) and by trial and error. Experience proved the usefulness of citrus fruits in the prevention and treatment of scurvy more than two centuries before the discovery of vitamin C (or controlled trials of treatment). An effective treatment for pernicious anemia (liver extract) was devised decades before the discovery of vitamin B_{12}. Effective treatments for epilepsy have been found without any good understanding of its cause. The best rationale for electroconvulsive therapy in depression is that it is often effective. Clearly, when a treatment is extremely useful, as in some of these examples, controlled trials may either be unnecessary, or very brief. Unfortunately, no treatment used for MS to this date falls in this category.

Until the exact cause of MS is discovered, there will certainly remain a place for a trial of treatments that may be partially effective, and whose only good rationale is that they may work. Pilot studies of such agents are appropriate, and, if positive, they should be subjected to controlled trial to determine that they are indeed effective. This is especially important if the treatment has potentially serious side-effects, or if it is very expensive.

This chapter contains a description of more than 50 treatments that have been claimed to be of benefit. The rationale for many of them is nonexistent or weak, based on current scientific principles and what we now know about MS. Only a few have had a controlled trial.

Why have not all of the methods presented in this chapter been subjected to a scientific controlled trial? The reasons are varied. In some instances the treatments were advocated years ago, before such trials were standardized. Another reason may be that some advocates are so convinced, they believe a trial would be unethical. A more likely reason is that controlled trials are expensive and time-consuming, often requiring 2 years or more for each agent. Therefore, physicians doing research on MS tend to spend their time where the rationale seems most sound, and the likelihood of success the greatest.

Some of the methods outlined in this chapter have clearly been the subject of commercial exploitation. Unfortunately, there are many instances in which clinics promote a specific "treatment" that is, in fact, of unproven value. Such institutions thrive on the very natural frustration and, frequently, the desperation of MS patients, and exploit the high likelihood of a placebo response in patients who have faith and believe they will be helped. Rumor and the international spread of anecdotes of success maintain the reputation of many such clinics.

There is no doubt that an appropriate combination of physical and spiritual activity can do much to stimulate a positive coping attitude in MS patients as well as improvement in the activities of daily living. The problem is to differentiate an unethical operation from a professional one. The Therapeutic Claims Committee advocates that MS patients respond to new therapeutic claims only if (a) participation is undertaken in consultation with their regular physicians, and (b) if the cost of treatment does not strain their financial resources.

MISCELLANEOUS EMPIRICAL TREATMENTS: INJECTED MATERIALS

Intravenous Yeasts (Proper-myl)

Description: A preparation of cells from three species of yeast, administered intravenously.

Rationale: It has been claimed that Proper-myl augments bodily defenses against infections and allergic reactions. It may be expected to act biologically much like typhoid vaccine.

Evaluation: As is often true, early reports were encouraging, but later reports showed results no better than known ineffective "treatments" for MS.

Risk/Costs: Occasional mild fever.

Conclusion: On the basis of published data, Proper-myl appears to be ineffective in the treatment of MS.

In the opinion of the Committee, there appears to be no generally accepted scientific basis for use of this therapy. It has never been tested in a proper controlled trial. Risks are undetermined.

MISCELLANEOUS EMPIRICAL TREATMENTS: INJECTED MATERIALS

Pancreatic Extract (Depropanex)

Description: A preparation derived from beef pancreas, given intramuscularly. The exact composition is not known, but it does not contain protein.

Rationale: Depropanex was used in MS treatment because it was considered to have both a vasodilating effect and an influence on carbohydrate metabolism.

Evaluation: In a small uncontrolled series, most patients were considered improved, whereas one was unchanged and one patient worsened. Improvement was chiefly in speech, spasticity, and general feeling of well-being, but was not very impressive. Progression was not prevented.

Risks/Costs: Foreign large molecules, if injected repeatedly, may induce severe, sometimes life-threatening reactions.

Conclusion: On the basis of the limited data, this treatment cannot be considered effective in MS.

In the opinion of the Committee, this therapy has been adequately tested and shown to be without value. Risks are undetermined.

MISCELLANEOUS EMPIRICAL TREATMENTS: INJECTED MATERIALS

Heart and Pancreas Extract (Pancorphen)

Description: A weak protein solution prepared by digesting beef heart with hog pancreas. It was used as a culture medium for growing bacteria.

Rationale: A similar culture medium had been used to grow bacteria in the preparation of a vaccine used to treat MS in 1930 (Purves-Stewart vaccine). It was suggested much later that the "success" of the Purves-Stewart vaccine was due to the culture medium, although the vaccine had long been shown to be ineffective.

Evaluation: Pancorphen was administered intravenously. Immediate worsening of neurologic symptoms occurred and lasted varying times, from hours to 2 weeks.

Risk/Costs: In addition to worsening of neurologic symptoms, general symptoms of fatigue, shortness of breath, hives, edema, and eczema occurred.

Conclusion: Pancorphen appears unacceptable as a treatment for MS.

In the opinion of the Committee, this therapy should not be used because of reported harmful effects.

MISCELLANEOUS EMPIRICAL TREATMENTS: INJECTED MATERIALS

Snake Venom (PROven, Venogen, Horvi MS9)

Description: PROven is a processed mixture of cobra, krait, and water moccasin venoms for subcutaneous injection. It has had spectrographic analysis, but its exact composition is not established. It appears to contain many proteins and some of the numerous enzymatic activities of the original venoms used in the mixture.

Rationale: The original idea for using snake venom in MS treatment occurred when a person who worked with snakes was bitten by a krait. Among the neurologic symptoms he suffered were some that suggested stimulation of the nervous system. Subsequently, there were many additional suggestions: that PROven might act as an immune stimulant, might prevent the action of a slow or persistent virus, or might act because of the nerve growth factor which it contains. Claims are also made that PROven reduces inflammation and pain. None of these suggestions has been investigated scientifically. PROven has also been suggested as a treatment for arthritis and for lupus, herpes simplex, herpes zoster, muscular dystrophy, Parkinson's disease, myasthenia gravis, and amyotrophic lateral sclerosis.

Evaluation: Patients receive 20 injections initially and continue the injections at home. The follow-up is chiefly by letters or phone calls from patients who feel they've been helped. There is no attempt to seek out patients who have not shown improvement. There have been no reports of objective or quantified examination to document any changes. The Food and Drug Administration has banned the sale of snake venom for the treatment of MS and arthritis until it is tested for safety and effectiveness. PROven continues to be dispensed by several Florida physicians. A similar mixture known as Horvi MS9 (or Horvi Psy 4 or Harviton) is sold in drugstores in Germany. An earlier mixture, Venogen, is no longer on the market.

Risks/Costs: Pain and swelling are induced at the injection site. These tend to diminish as the injections are repeated over days to weeks. One bad allergic reaction to PROven has been reported. One young woman receiving PROven injections died with an unusual type of brain hemorrhage; it could not be determined if this was due to the treatment.

Conclusion: There are no objective controlled studies. The lack of standardized preparation of known composition and proven safety precludes clinical trials at this time. Based on the evidence examined, this treatment is not recommended.

In the opinion of the Committee, there appears to be no generally accepted scientific basis for use of this therapy. It has never been tested in a proper controlled trial. Its use carries significant risk.

MISCELLANEOUS EMPIRICAL TREATMENTS: INJECTED MATERIALS

Octacosanol

Description: A simple long-chain alcohol.

Rationale: The use of octacosanol is based on the idea that in MS there is a disturbance in the incorporation of long-chain fatty acids into myelin lipids, and the suggestion that the corresponding long-chain alcohols might stimulate this process and thus correct the problem or perhaps accelerate repair of damaged myelin.

Evaluation: Daily administration of octacosanol in several dozen MS patients is said to have led to continued improvement in two of three, and remission of symptoms over a few days or weeks in about 10%. The treatment is also said to arrest the unrelated disease ALS in 75% of cases, and claims have been made that octacosanol is effective in the treatment of muscular atrophy, myasthenia gravis, amyotonia congenita, several types of cerebral palsy, brain damage, poststroke syndrome, myositis (inflammation of voluntary muscle), dermatomyositis, and several other neuromuscular disorders. The findings depend on clinical impressions rather than quantified objective study. There has not been a controlled study, and the degree of improvement observed is comparable to that seen with treatments regarded today as ineffective.

Risks/Costs: Negligible.

Conclusion: There is no objective evidence at the present time that this treatment is of value in MS.

In the opinion of the Committee, there appears to be no generally accepted scientific basis for use of this therapy. It has never been tested in a proper controlled trial. Risks are undetermined.

MISCELLANEOUS EMPIRICAL TREATMENTS: INJECTED MATERIALS

Superoxide Dismutase (Orgotein; Orgosein; Palosein)

Description: Superoxide dismutase (SOD) is a metalloprotein enzyme that combines with and "neutralizes" free radicals of oxygen (superoxides) appearing as a normal toxic byproduct of cellular metabolism. It is available in health food stores as an extract of liver in tablet form and is used in veterinary practice as an antiinflammatory agent (by injection).

Rationale: The theory has been developed that tissue superoxides may be involved in the "hardening" of connective tissue in some forms of chronic inflammation and in tissue degeneration and aging. Theoretically, augmenting the supply of SOD, which would be presumed to reduce the level of superoxides, would reduce inflammation and lessen these toxic effects.

Evaluation: SOD has been widely advertised as useful in a variety of inflammatory and sclerotic conditions. It has been shown, when injected, to be safe and effective in reducing inflammation after radiation and tissue damage of the joints, bladder, and bowel. There are unsubstantiated claims of its usefulness in rheumatoid arthritis and multiple sclerosis. Because proteins are denatured and digested in the stomach, it is doubtful that this substance would remain biologically active after oral use. In one uncontrolled trial of 23 MS patients, the results could not be differentiated from those expected in a placebo response. In a recent "controlled, double-blind" study of 200 patients given orgotein or a placebo over a year's time, with further observation for two years, no attempt was made to obtain objective data by scoring the severity of disease or counting the actual number of relapses; yet the claim was made that all treated patients improved, three quarters of them resumed work, and flare-ups of MS were eliminated.

Risks/Costs: SOD is apparently not toxic.

Conclusion: From available reports, there appears to be no published evidence that SOD is effective in MS.

In the opinion of the Committee, there appears to be no generally accepted scientific basis for use of this therapy. It has never been tested in a proper controlled trial. Risks are undetermined.

MISCELLANEOUS EMPIRICAL TREATMENTS: INJECTED MATERIALS

Procaine Hydrochloride

Description: Procaine is a simple chemical with anesthetic properties. KH3 is the proprietary name for a procaine compound in capsule form available by prescription in limited areas of the United States and in Europe. It is said to improve physical and mental efficiency and has been recommended for treatment of the depression of old age.

Rationale: Procaine is used in local surgery, and in skin creams for treatment of local burns (sunburn, etc.). There is no known basis for its use in the treatment of MS.

Evaluation: No evaluation of KH3 has been conducted for MS because there is no clinical indication for its use. Scattered anecdotal reports of treatment have led to clinical effects that cannot be differentiated from the placebo response.

Risks/Costs: The material is not approved for use by the U.S. Food and Drug Administration. There are no risks except in rare cases of procaine allergy.

Conclusion: There appears to be no present indication for the use of procaine in MS.

In the opinion of the Committee, there appears to be no generally accepted scientific basis for use of this therapy. It has never been tested in a proper controlled trial. Its use carries significant risk.

MISCELLANEOUS EMPIRICAL TREATMENTS: INJECTED MATERIALS

Dimethyl Sulfoxide

Description: Dimethyl sulfoxide (DMSO) is a potent solvent for chemicals and has been widely used in industry as a degreaser.

Rationale: Because of its rapid absorption by skin and its qualities as a liniment, DMSO has been used for the treatment of sprains and muscle pains in animals. It is under study, in purified form, for oral or intravenous administration or administration by way of the skin, to determine whether it can help transport drugs more effectively into tissue cells for treatment of specific diseases. In animal studies, it has been shown to be immunosuppressive, and research is under way to determine its possible usefulness in treatment of autoimmune diseases. DMSO is approved by the U.S. Food and Drug Administration for administration into the bladder in a 50% solution for therapy of an uncommon intractable form of chronic inflammation.

Evaluation: DMSO has achieved some notoriety as a nonprescription drug for the "treatment" of arthritis and other chronic handicapping diseases. There is no evidence at this time that it provides a predictable change in the clinical severity of any of these conditions beyond what can be explained by the placebo response. There has been no controlled study of DMSO in MS.

Risks/Costs: The rapid rate of absorption carries the danger of absorbing toxic contaminants (if "industrial grade" is used). Side-effects include rashes, nausea, vomiting, chills, drowsiness, and a characteristic garlic odor on the breath. DMSO is relatively inexpensive, and is available as a nonprescription item in health stores, hardware stores, and various other outlets.

Conclusion: There is no acceptable medical evidence to support the use of DMSO in MS at the present time.

In the opinion of the Committee, there appears to be no generally accepted scientific basis for use of this therapy. It has never been tested in a proper controlled trial. Risks are undetermined.

MISCELLANEOUS EMPIRICAL TREATMENTS: INJECTED MATERIALS

Alphasal (formerly Cholorazone or Vitamin X)

Description: A product of electrolysis of a saline solution. If used immediately, contains ozone. Taken orally or by injection.

Rationale: This product was developed in Greece and has been recommended for prophylaxis or treatment of many diseases. The rationale for its use is obscure.

Evaluation: Only anecdotal information is available. More than 500 individuals with 50 different diseases are said to have been treated, under the supervision of the inventor. Positive results were obtained in all 50 and "cures" in 30, including MS, arthritis, and cancer. No controlled studies have been done.

Risks/Costs: Unknown.

Conclusion: No scientifically acceptable evidence exists for the usefulness of alphasal in MS.

In the opinion of the Committee, there appears to be no generally accepted scientific basis for use of this therapy. It has never been tested in a proper controlled trial. Risks are undetermined.

MISCELLANEOUS EMPIRICAL TREATMENTS: INJECTED MATERIALS

Cellular Therapy

Description: Injection of ground-up brain or other tissues freshly prepared from unborn calves, lambs, or pigs.

Rationale: A Swiss clinic developed this approach more than 40 years ago for the treatment of a wide variety of diseases. Injection of fetal tissue corresponding to the diseased tissue of the patient was supposed to bring new vigor and fight disease in that tissue. This is not regarded seriously today as a scientific theory.

Evaluation: Many patients with MS were treated with fetal brain. Improvement was claimed in the majority of patients on the basis of subjective impressions. No controlled studies were ever done.

Risks/Costs: Two cases were reported in which the injections produced autoimmunization, and the patients developed EAE comparable to the experimental disease in laboratory animals. One death owing to this "treatment" has been reported.

Conclusion: What little published information is available suggests that this treatment should be considered ineffective in MS and potentially dangerous.

In the opinion of the Committee, there appears to be no generally accepted scientific basis for use of this therapy. It has never been tested in a proper controlled trial. Its use carries significant risk.

MISCELLANEOUS EMPIRICAL TREATMENTS: INJECTED MATERIALS

Allergens

Description: Repeated injections of food or other allergens, used in desensitization for asthma and hay fever.

Rationale: This treatment was based on the theory that MS might be an allergic reaction to common environmental substances.

Evaluation: There have been attempts to identify environmental allergens, including foods, that might play a role in the MS process. This was followed by attempts to affect the clinical course of MS by desensitization with increasing injections of the allergen. Elimination diets have also been tried. There is no convincing evidence that these measures influenced the course of the disease.

Risks/Costs: Negligible risks. Cost of repeated injections is significant.

Conclusion: All available data suggest that this treatment should be considered ineffective in MS.

In the opinion of the Committee, there appears to be no generally accepted scientific basis for use of this therapy. It has never been tested in a proper controlled trial. It is relatively free of serious adverse side-effects during long-term use. It is very expensive.

MISCELLANEOUS EMPIRICAL TREATMENTS: INJECTED MATERIALS

Rodilemid

Description: A mixture of chelating (metal-binding) agents, developed in Rumania. It includes L-cysteine, the calcium sodium salt of ethylenediamine tetraacetic acid (EDTA), and calcium gluconate. It is taken as a series of six daily intramuscular injections at intervals of 1–4 months.

Rationale: This mixture was developed to "facilitate calcium penetration into the neuron" and thus "inhibit viral infection." It is said not to lower body or cell calcium and thus lacks the toxicity associated with chelation therapy. No studies have been done of possible direct effects on nerve conduction or antiinflammatory action on lymphocytes or macrophages.

Evaluation: In a long-term uncontrolled study, it is claimed that Rodilemid therapy gave lasting improvement (at least one point on the Kurtzke scale) in 80% of patients with chronic progressive or clinically stable MS. These results are unconfirmed thus far.

Risks/Costs: Toxicity appears to be low.

Conclusion: Rodilemid is unproven as a therapy for MS.

In the opinion of the Committee, there appears to be no generally accepted scientific basis for use of this therapy. It has never been tested in a proper controlled trial. Risks are undetermined.

MISCELLANEOUS EMPIRICAL TREATMENTS: INJECTED MATERIALS

Autogenous Vaccine

Description: Vaccine prepared from bacteria growing in or on the patient's own body.

Rationale: Such vaccines were used a half century ago on the old theory that various diseases might be "allergic" reactions to the individual's own bacteria.

Evaluation: No controlled trials have ever been carried out in MS, nor is there any accepted basis for such trials at present. Some reports indicate that the treatment is dangerous.

Risks/Costs: Not commercially available, and costs undetermined.

Conclusion: Bacterial products may be IFN inducers, including IFN gamma. Because of this and lack of controlled studies, this treatment should not be used.

In the opinion of the Committee, this therapy should not be used because of reported harmful effects.

MISCELLANEOUS EMPIRICAL TREATMENTS: INJECTED MATERIALS

Proneut

Description: A combination of measle vaccine, influenza vaccine, and histamine phosphate, the dose being individually determined for each patient.

Rationale: Proneut is used experimentally as a type of "provocation therapy" or "provocation-neutralization therapy" in MS treatment, using three components suspected of being the causative agent in MS. The patient receives repeated subcutaneous doses of the mixture.

Evaluation: The use of Proneut has been limited to subjective observations in an uncontrolled series of MS patients, with no attempt at full neurologic evaluation. The results reported are compatible with a placebo effect.

Risks/Costs: A high fee is charged for a simple mixture, which patients are taught to administer themselves.

Conclusion: There appears to be no convincing evidence at present that this treatment is effective in MS.

In the opinion of the Committee, there appears to be no generally accepted scientific basis for use of this therapy. It has never been tested in a proper controlled trial. Risks are undetermined. It is very expensive.

MISCELLANEOUS EMPIRICAL TREATMENTS: INJECTED MATERIALS

Alpha-Fetoprotein (α-Fetoprotein)

Description: Alpha-fetoprotein (AFP) is a protein produced by the liver of the fetus in the womb to protect it against the mother's immune system. It has been purified and used experimentally.

Rationale: The severity of MS sometimes diminishes during late pregnancy, the time when the fetus is producing large amounts of AFP. Experimentally, AFP is effective in suppressing EAE. It, therefore, may be of interest for trial in MS.

Evaluation: A trial of AFP in MS is under consideration at the present time.

Risks/Costs: Unknown.

Conclusion: None, at present.

In the opinion of the Committee, there appears to be no generally accepted scientific basis for use of this therapy. It has never been tested in a proper controlled trial. Risks are undetermined.

MISCELLANEOUS EMPIRICAL TREATMENTS: INJECTED MATERIALS

Immunoglobulins (Gamma Globulin)

Description: Immunoglobulins are the antibody-containing fraction of human plasma. They are usually injected intramuscularly.

Rationale: Transfer (by injection) of pooled immunoglobulin from many donors transfers antibodies to a variety of viruses, bacteria, and other infectious agents. This is highly effective, for example, in preventing hepatitis-A virus infection. It has also been suggested that artificially sustained high levels of circulating gamma globulin may block the harmful action of antibodies (which are also gamma globulin) active in the MS patients, for example, antibodies against myelin.

Evaluation: Pooled human gamma globulin given over a period of 6 months showed no benefit to a series of treated MS patients as compared with controls. Intraglobin, a concentrated, chemically modified gamma globulin that can be given intravenously, has been given in high dose at 2-month intervals during 1 year to 20 patients with the exacerbating–remitting type of MS. The patients showed a slight decrease in relapse rate and a decrease in the average severity of their clinical disease as compared with their own pretreatment record. This change may correspond simply to the natural history of the disease.

Risks/Costs: Injection of pooled gamma globulin carries almost no risks, other than transient pain at the injection site. There is current concern in the literature over the possibility that gamma globulin may carry AIDS. Gamma globulin is expensive.

Conclusion: On the basis of the published results, this treatment appears to be ineffective in MS.

In the opinion of the Committee, there appears to be no generally accepted scientific basis for use of this therapy. It has never been tested in a proper controlled trial. Its use carries significant risk. It is very expensive.

MISCELLANEOUS EMPIRICAL TREATMENTS: INJECTED MATERIALS

Immunobiological Revitalization

Description: Purified rabbit antibodies against human bone marrow, spleen, and thymus, supplemented by an undefined "human placental product."

Rationale: A Russian scientist, Bogomoletz, originally described the use of antibody against lymphoid tissues (so-called "antireticulo-cytotoxic" antibody) as a stimulant to immune function, when the antibody was given in repeated low doses.

Evaluation: This treatment was widely used in the U.S.S.R. before World War II and has since spread to the rest of the world. As "immunobiological revitalization," it is said to cure diseases affecting all systems of the body including allergies, cancer, and mental disease, and to improve sexuality, extend life span, and provide beneficial cosmetic effects. These claims have been made for MS as well; 38 patients were treated between 1974 and 1979. No objective observations were made to substantiate the claim.

Risks/Costs: The treatment is usually offered as part of a broad and expensive "program." Risks are unknown.

Conclusion: Based on the evidence examined, this treatment is not recommended.

In the opinion of the Committee, there appears to be no generally accepted scientific basis for use of this therapy. It has never been tested in a proper controlled trial. Risks are undetermined. It is very expensive.

MISCELLANEOUS EMPIRICAL TREATMENTS: INJECTED MATERIALS

Proteolytic Enzymes

Description: A mixture of digestive enzymes (pancreatin, chymotrypsin, and several others), given intravenously in repeated dosage.

Rationale: A mixture of proteolytic enzymes is reported to have therapeutic action in inflammatory diseases caused by immune complexes (antigen–antibody aggregates), such as glomerulonephritis and rheumatoid arthritis, as well as in coagulative disorders. Immune complex formation may possibly play a role in lesion formation in acute MS.

Evaluation: A standardized commercial system enzyme mixture has been used in 80 MS patients for more than 5 years, in a preliminary study carried out in Austria. With early high-dose administration, acute attacks are reported to be aborted in some cases. With long-term treatment, it is claimed that further attacks and progression are prevented in 50% of the patients. The treatment, however, is relatively ineffective in patients already treated for some time with azathioprine, ACTH, or corticosteroids. Plans are being developed for controlled studies.

Risks/Costs: This therapy is said to be essentially nontoxic. However, any intravenous injection, especially with foreign proteins, carries substantial potential risks. The cost of repetitive intravenous therapy is usually high.

Conclusion: Inadequate published information exists to permit informed judgment about this therapy.

In the opinion of the Committee, there appears to be no generally accepted scientific basis for use of this therapy. It has never been tested in a proper controlled trial. Risks are undetermined.

MISCELLANEOUS EMPIRICAL TREATMENTS: INJECTED MATERIALS AND ORAL ADMINISTRATION

Calcium Orotate; Calcium Aminoethyl Phosphate

Description: Calcium orotate and calcium aminoethyl phosphate (AEP) are calcium salts of synthetic organic compounds, given intravenously and by mouth.

Rationale: These substances were developed to facilitate the carrying of calcium, and making it more available for body metabolism.

Evaluation: Both compounds have been used for over 16 years in a clinic in West Germany for the treatment of conditions considered to be inflammatory or autoimmune in nature. The treatment, especially calcium AEP, is said to have a very favorable effect on 5–78% of patients with MS. Objective and quantified data are not available, and there is no documented proof that therapies of this sort produce any benefit. They are clearly the subject of considerable commercial exploitation.

Risks/Costs: There are said to be no significant side-effects. Costs are high.

Conclusion: In the absence of a properly designed clinical study, the claim of favorable effect remains undocumented.

In the opinion of the Committee, there appears to be no generally accepted scientific basis for use of this therapy. It has never been tested in a proper controlled trial. It is relatively free of serious adverse side-effects during long-term use. It is very expensive.

MISCELLANEOUS EMPIRICAL TREATMENTS: ORAL ADMINISTRATION

Oral Calcium + Magnesium + Vitamin D

Description: Inexpensive chemicals available commercially, taken by mouth.

Rationale: Epidemiologic studies suggested a correlation of MS prevalence with restricted intake of calcium, magnesium, and vitamin D. This observation is supported by the finding of abnormal calcium and magnesium levels in MS patients' serum. Finally, because both minerals are essential to the myelination process, deficiency is thought to produce instability of myelin.

Evaluation: In a small preliminary trial, patients were fed calcium, magnesium, and vitamin D for a period of 1 to 2 years. They experienced fewer relapses of MS during the period of treatment than would be expected from their histories. However, because the frequency of relapses in individual patients tends to diminish with time, this observation is difficult to interpret. A larger, controlled study is being planned.

Risks/Costs: Negligible.

Conclusion: The efficacy of this treatment is as yet undocumented.

In the opinion of the Committee, there appears to be no generally accepted scientific basis for use of this therapy. It has never been tested in a proper controlled trial. Risks are undetermined.

MISCELLANEOUS EMPIRICAL TREATMENTS: INJECTED MATERIALS AND ORAL ADMINISTRATION

Sodium Bicarbonate, Phosphates

Description: Simple chemicals, given intravenously (sodium bicarbonate) or by mouth (phosphates).

Rationale: Experimental studies suggested that nerve fiber conduction would be improved by decreasing the concentration of calcium available to demyelinated fibers.

Evaluation: In clinical trials, it has been possible to reduce calcium levels temporarily by giving intravenous sodium bicarbonate or large oral doses of phosphates, both of which bind calcium. These trials resulted in rapid but temporary measurable improvement in a number of neurologic defects. Continued use of such agents and long-term low calcium levels are not compatible with continued health. Therefore, these agents are not satisfactory treatments for MS. The studies do demonstrate that nerve fiber conduction can be favorably altered by chemical means, and encourage the search for agents that can be used over extended periods.

Risks/Costs: Long-term use is not compatible with good health.

Conclusion: These substances are not recommended as treatments.

In the opinion of the Committee, there appears to be no generally accepted scientific basis for use of this therapy. It has never been tested in a proper controlled trial. Risks are undetermined.

MISCELLANEOUS EMPIRICAL TREATMENTS: INJECTED MATERIALS

Chelation Therapy with Ethylenediamine Tetraacetic Acid

Description: A simple chemical that chelates (binds) metals very efficiently and is used in cases of lead poisoning to remove lead from the body. Must be injected intravenously over several hours.

Rationale: Several practitioners have advocated the use of "chelation therapy" for MS, along with a wide variety of other diseases including cancer, Parkinson's disease, arthritis, heart attacks, and strokes, as well as simpler problems such as leg cramps, poor vision, senility, poor memory, etc.

Evaluation: The Food and Drug Administration, the Veterans Administration, and other professional associations are unanimous in calling "chelation therapy" worthless for the purposes claimed. The Harvard Medical School Health Letter concludes: "There is no credible evidence that chelation therapy works as claimed . . . except as an elaborate placebo."

Risks/Costs: This "therapy" is "potentially" lethal without adequate supervision. It was implicated by Federal officials in 14 deaths at one clinic. Costs may run as high as $6,000 for treatment extending over several months.

Conclusion: Chelation therapy for MS is not based on acceptable published evidence, and is dangerous.

In the opinion of the Committee, there appears to be no generally accepted scientific basis for use of this therapy. It has never been tested in a proper controlled trial. Its use carries significant risk. It is very expensive.

MISCELLANEOUS EMPIRICAL TREATMENTS: ORAL ADMINISTRATION

Hyperimmune Colostrum (Immune Milk)

Description: Pregnant cows are inoculated with measles vaccine or other viruses considered to be possibly related to MS. Colostrum (early milk), collected by veterinarians from these cows during the first 2 days after delivery, is frozen for preservation and subsequently taken by mouth.

Rationale: In humans, antibodies pass across the placenta from the mother's circulation into the circulation of the baby, providing it with immunity against a variety of infections before birth. In cattle, antibodies do not pass across the placenta, but pass from the mother to the newborn calf in the colostrum during nursing. The use of hyperimmune bovine colostrum as a treatment for MS is based on evidence that one or more viruses may be associated with the development of MS.

Evaluation: No studies have been done to determine whether there are antibodies to the vaccines used in the serum of the cows, in the colostrum, or in the patients. Bovine antibodies in general are not absorbed by adult humans from the stomach or intestine. A sizable number of patients with MS in various parts of the United States have received hyperimmune bovine colostrum. The responses of patients were obtained by questionnaire, and improvement was reported by a majority. However, much of the improvement related to stamina, well-being, pain, and activity level.

In a preliminary double-blind, crossover study of 12 MS patients, three showed some worsening when taken off immune colostrum; two of these had very mild disease to start with.

In a pilot Japanese study, published in 1984, most MS patients given immune colostrum containing measles antibody "improved," whereas most patients in a smaller group given normal colostrum worsened. No data are provided as to duration or severity of disease or the possible occurrence of exacerbations in individual patients and there was no matching or randomization of test and control groups.

Risks/Costs: The cost of hyperimmune colostrum appears to be modest. A few patients reported skin rash, "mild allergic reaction," or not feeling well.

Conclusion: This treatment remains unproven, and is not recommended. A clinical trial of adequate size would be required to determine whether it has any value.

In the opinion of the Committee, there appears to be no generally accepted scientific basis for use of this therapy. It has never been tested in a proper controlled trial. Risks are undetermined.

MISCELLANEOUS EMPIRICAL TREATMENTS: ORAL ADMINISTRATION

Metabolic Therapy

Description: A complex program of regimens and medications said to affect mineral balance, diet (both how much and what is in it), and bowel function, e.g., alkalinity of the small intestine; also immune colostrum and high doses of vitamin C (as "antiviral agents"), SOD, vitamin A, "thymotropic" tablets to "stimulate the immune system," octacosanol, B complex vitamins.

Rationale: The components of this program are discussed individually elsewhere in this volume.

Evaluation: "Metabolic therapy" has never been subjected to a scientifically planned clinical trial in which objective measurements of effect can be determined. As noted in discussion elsewhere in this volume, the Committee is aware of no scientific basis for any of the components of this program. Various forms of "metabolic therapy" have been advocated as cures for cancer and arthritis, with poor evidence of effectiveness.

Risks/Costs: Vitamins A and C in large doses produce toxic side effects. Costs are substantial.

Conclusion: This is an unproven, expensive, and possibly dangerous procedure with no known scientific basis.

In the opinion of the Committee, there appears to be no generally accepted scientific basis for use of this therapy. It has never been tested in a proper controlled trial. Long-term use may be associated with significant serious side-effects. It is very expensive.

MISCELLANEOUS EMPIRICAL TREATMENTS: ORAL ADMINISTRATION

Promazine Hydrochloride (Sparine)

Description: A phenothiazine drug.

Rationale: The hypothesis is offered that specific immune responses to acute viral infection are accompanied by blood–brain barrier damage. Drugs that antagonize a "pressor" effect during the prodromal phase that precedes exacerbations are thought to abort the disease process.

Evaluation: Evidence to support the use of Sparine is entirely anecdotal. No controlled trials have been carried out. Other drugs said to have similar effects, on similar anecdotal grounds, include oxprenolol, propranolol, and Largactil.

Risks/Costs: Negligible.

Conclusion: The value of phenothiazine and related drugs in aborting MS exacerbations remains to be established.

In the opinion of the Committee, there appears to be no generally accepted scientific basis for use of this therapy. It has never been tested in a proper controlled trial. Long-term use may be associated with significant serious side-effects.

MISCELLANEOUS EMPIRICAL TREATMENTS: ORAL ADMINISTRATION

Le Gac Therapy

Description: Treatment with broad-spectrum antibiotics (Terramycin, Aureomycin), combined with hot baths.

Rationale: MS is attributed to infection with rickettsiae, infectious agents intermediate between bacteria and viruses. In one study, antibodies to rickettsiae were found more frequently in MS patients than in a series of controls. Use of broad-spectrum antibiotics is intended to cure such infection.

Evaluation: No epidemiologic or bacteriological evidence to relate MS to rickettsial infection has ever been obtained. MS patients show more frequent and higher antibody levels than controls to a variety of infectious agents, probably as a consequence of faulty immune regulation. The Le Gac treatment has been supported by a series of anecdotal cases in which patients, usually treated during an acute attack of MS, subsequently improved. No controlled trial of the therapy has ever been done.

Risks/Costs: Negligible. Hot baths may cause transient or even permanent worsening of symptoms in some patients.

Conclusion: Based on evidence examined, this treatment is not recommended.

In the opinion of the Committee, there appears to be no generally accepted scientific basis for use of this therapy. It has never been tested in a proper controlled trial. Its use carries significant risk.

MISCELLANEOUS EMPIRICAL TREATMENTS: ORAL ADMINISTRATION

Nystatin

Description: An antifungal agent, particularly effective against yeast infections *(Candida albicans)*, usually employed with a yeast-free, low carbohydrate diet.

Rationale: Two physicians have tried to relate a variety of chronic disorders to overgrowth of *Candida albicans* in the intestinal tract, after use of carbohydrate-rich diets, birth control pills, steroids, or other antibiotics. MS is included, along with schizophrenia, depression, psoriasis, arthritis, headache, premenstrual tension, and various other nervous system disorders.

Evaluation: There is no widely accepted scientific or medical evidence that any of the above conditions is related to candidiasis. Evidence for efficacy of nystatin in MS is largely anecdotal. Rigorous controlled studies have not been reported.

Risks/Costs: Modest.

Conclusion: Use of nystatin in MS is not recommended.

In the opinion of the Committee, there appears to be no generally accepted scientific basis for use of this therapy. It has never been tested in a proper controlled trial. It is relatively free of serious adverse side-effects during short-term use.

MISCELLANEOUS EMPIRICAL TREATMENTS: PHYSICAL AND SURGICAL MANIPULATIONS

Acupuncture

Description: Acupuncture is a 4,000-year-old Chinese procedure that has been known to the Western world since the 1600s. It is performed by inserting fine needles into specific skin sites in the expectation of influencing the function of underlying organs. Twirling, vibrating, or electrically stimulating the needles is considered to enhance the effectiveness of the procedure.

Rationale: Acupuncture has been used extensively for relief of pain of various origins. It appears to be associated with increased endorphin activity (natural morphine-like substances in the CNS). The use of acupuncture might serve for relief of pain and muscle spasm.

Evaluation: There is anecdotal evidence that some patients treated with acupuncture feel better. There is no evidence that progression of the disease is slowed or relapses prevented. Changes in bladder function have been observed, but these may be due to the highly variable natural course of bladder symptoms.

Risks/Costs: Any procedure involving penetration of the skin by needles may carry the risk of hepatitis. Cost of any repeated procedure is significant.

Conclusion: Based on the evidence examined, this treatment is considered to have no effect on the disease process in MS, and has not been shown to have any value in the symptomatic management of patients with disease. Some patients may experience temporary relief of pain.

In the opinion of the Committee, there appears to be no generally accepted scientific basis for use of this therapy. It has never been tested in a proper controlled trial. Long-term use may be associated with significant serious side-effects. It is very expensive.

MISCELLANEOUS EMPIRICAL TREATMENTS: PHYSICAL AND SURGICAL MANIPULATIONS

Dorsal Column Stimulation

Description: The dorsal columns of the spinal cord are large bundles of nerve fibers that carry the sense of touch and the sense of position from the legs, trunk, and arms up to the brain. The spinal cord is protected by a connective tissue wrapping, known as dura. Electrical stimulation of the dorsal columns requires implantation of two electrodes on the overlying dura. This formerly necessitated an open operation, but is now done by passing the electrodes through a special needle. The electrodes are connected with an implanted stimulator or radio receiver.

Rationale: The use of dorsal column stimulation (DCS) in MS began empirically when the procedure was used with an MS patient to control pain, and it was noted that the patient functioned better after sessions of stimulation. Subsequently it was claimed that DCS favorably altered the functioning of the neural circuits of the CNS, especially the spinal cord and brainstem, and produced measurable changes in evoked potentials and in both subjective state and objective neurologic function in some patients.

Evaluation: Claims are made of benefit from DCS in a variety of diseases. These include athetosis, cerebral palsy, dystonia, posttraumatic and poststroke spasticity, epilepsy, and "degenerative disease." In one series of 300 such cases, 70–85% were said to have shown improvement in one or another neural function. However, in at least four series of MS cases in which there was careful neurologic follow-up, a few patients showed initial subjective improvement but none showed either subjective or objective benefit at the end of 2 years and most had abandoned the treatment.

Risks/Costs: Infection, hemorrhage, and serious spinal cord injury have occurred in a small proportion of patients. Slipping of electrodes out of place or breakage of electrode wires occurs in up to 65% of the cases. This requires an operation to replace or remove electrodes. In a small proportion of cases, the operation may be complicated by hemorrhage at the operative site, spinal cord compression, and paraplegia (total paralysis) of the lower limbs. The costs include surgical fees, operation room costs, and hospitalization, which may amount to more than $25,000 and usually are not reimbursable by third-party carriers.

Conclusion: This procedure is ineffective and dangerous. The costs and the risks are high. It is not recommended for use in patients with MS.

In the opinion of the Committee, this therapy should not be used because of reported harmful effects. Its use carries significant risk. It is very expensive.

MISCELLANEOUS EMPIRICAL TREATMENTS: PHYSICAL AND SURGICAL MANIPULATIONS

Hyperbaric Oxygen

Description: Breathing oxygen under increased pressure in a specially constructed chamber.

Rationale: Hyperbaric oxygen (HBO) has been used effectively in burns, gas gangrene, and air embolism. It has been reported to improve mental functions of aged patients. Early reports suggested that HBO might produce temporary improvement in MS patients. HBO is also immunosuppressive and suppresses EAE, the animal model of MS. However, oxygen at normal pressure is also reported to suppress EAE.

Evaluation: HBO has been used over several years in the treatment of a considerable number of MS patients in the United States, United Kingdom, Italy, and the Soviet Union. In uncontrolled studies and in one controlled study, patients with chronic, progressive disease were reported to show significant improvement after a course of treatment lasting several weeks. They generally returned to pretreatment level some weeks after treatment was stopped, but would respond rapidly after "booster" exposure to HBO.

In the spring of 1985, the results of six separate, controlled, double-blind studies were reported, which mimicked in detail the techniques described earlier as effective, including (in one instance) monthly booster treatments extending over 6 months. Assessments made use of MRI and electrophysiologic techniques in addition to more conventional neurologic and laboratory procedures. These trials, carried out in the United States, United Kingdom, Canada, and The Netherlands, are unanimous that HBO is without effect on any objective parameter of the disease process, with the single exception of minimal bladder improvement in some patients.

Risks/Costs: The procedure entails high cost, because the equipment is expensive, skilled technicians are required, and there must be frequent repeated visits. Exposure to oxygen at higher pressures or for longer periods than those recommended may produce serious side effects in the nervous system, the most extreme being blindness or convulsive episodes. Such effects may be seen in a small percentage of patients even when they are correctly treated.

Conclusion: Large-scale, double-blind controlled studies have proven that HBO is ineffective as a treatment for MS.

In the opinion of the Committee, this therapy has been adequately tested and shown to be without value. Its use carries significant risk. It is very expensive.

MISCELLANEOUS EMPIRICAL TREATMENTS: PHYSICAL AND SURGICAL MANIPULATIONS

Transcutaneous Nerve Stimulation

Description: Transcutaneous nerve stimulation (TNS) is a procedure in which electrodes are placed on the surface of the skin over certain nerves and electrical stimulation is carried out. The dose, varied by varying frequency, pulse width, and intensity (amplitude), determines which nerve fibers are activated.

Rationale: The stimulation of the CNS from the periphery is thought to improve CNS performance generally. This is really a variant of acupuncture technique and in some ways resembles old-fashioned "counter-irritant" techniques (mustard plaster, etc.). The newest way of doing the same thing is use of a low-powered laser beam. Stimulation for 20–30 min gives objective pain relief, and this has been clearly related to release of morphine-like compounds within the CNS and CSF. TNS is sometimes used in conjunction with oral administration of the unnatural amino acid d-phenylalanine, which is claimed to have an endorphin (morphine-like) effect, and vitamin B_{12}.

Evaluation: Subjective improvement and reduced spasticity have been reported to an extent not seen in MS patients subjected to sham stimulation. TNS is also said to reduce cerebellar tremor. Insufficient information exists to permit evaluation of this "treatment," because quantitative objective data have not so far been reported.

Risks/Costs: Local skin irritation under an electrode may occur. TNS does not have the drawbacks of DCS as an invasive procedure.

Conclusion: Quantified studies are needed to establish whether therapy with TNS has any value.

In the opinion of the Committee, there appears to be no generally accepted scientific basis for use of this therapy. It has never been tested in a proper controlled trial. It is relatively free of serious adverse side-effects during long-term use.

MISCELLANEOUS EMPIRICAL TREATMENTS: PHYSICAL AND SURGICAL MANIPULATIONS

Thalamotomy; Thalamic Stimulation

Description: Destruction of part of the thalamus by surgical means. More recently, electrical stimulation of the thalamus by surgically implanted electrodes has been reported to have a similar effect.

Rationale: The thalamus is the name given to a central region in the upper part of the brain. It contributes to the control of movement. Tremor and certain other involuntary movements can be reduced or abolished by thalamotomy or thalamic stimulation, and this procedure is used in various neurologic diseases.

Evaluation: In MS, loss of coordination is often associated with tremor during use of the arms or legs. In patients with severe tremors, thalamotomy has been performed with relief of the tremor, but without effect on other neurologic defects. Patients were selected who had had tremor for at least 1 year, to be certain that it would not remit spontaneously. The tremor frequently recurs within a few years after the operation. Surgeons are currently turning away from thalamotomy because of the attendant risks, and implanting electrodes in the same part of the brain as a less dangerous means of controlling tremor.

Risks/Costs: The risks are those of complications attending any brain operation. Thalamotomy on one side may result in weakness of the arm and leg on the opposite side, disturbance of recent memory, or speech and language disturbance; these may be due to enlargement of the operative wound by bleeding, especially in patients with high blood pressure. There may also be exacerbation of the MS. Although unilateral thalamic lesions carry a modest risk, there is always a chance that MS will have damaged the other side of the thalamus. Under these circumstances the risk of serious disability is high. Bilateral thalamotomy frequently causes pseudobulbar palsy and results in severe speech and swallowing difficulties. Costs are very high, including surgeon's fees, operating room charges, and hospitalization.

Conclusion: Based on the evidence examined, thalamotomy (and possibly thalamic stimulation) offers the possibility of control of tremor in a very small number of carefully selected MS patients, but the beneficial effect is of limited duration and is associated with substantial risks.

In the opinion of the Committee, this therapy may have some efficacy, but the evidence is conflicting, and it must be regarded as investigational. Its use carries significant risk.

MISCELLANEOUS EMPIRICAL TREATMENTS: PHYSICAL AND SURGICAL MANIPULATIONS

Sympathectomy and Ganglionectomy

Description: Sympathetic nerves and ganglions supplying blood vessels to the head are surgically removed in an effort to increase blood supply to the CNS.

Rationale: A special division of the nervous system, called the autonomic nervous system, controls such bodily functions as intestinal motility, heart rate, blood pressure, and blood vessel tone. Its sympathetic component constricts while parasympathetic activity dilates blood vessels. The use of this technique is based on the scientifically unproven assumption that the MS process involves inadequacy of local blood supply in the brain and spinal cord.

Evaluation: In the past, numerous agents intended to affect blood vessels and blood supply to the nervous system have been tried in MS treatment. They have all been abandoned as ineffective. The reported results with sympathectomy were also inconclusive. Since 1938, the procedure has been given up as a treatment for MS.

Risks/Costs: Those associated with major surgery.

Conclusion: The limited available data suggest that this treatment should not be considered effective in MS.

In the opinion of the Committee, there appears to be no generally accepted scientific basis for use of this therapy. It has never been tested in a proper controlled trial. Its use carries significant risk. It is very expensive.

MISCELLANEOUS EMPIRICAL TREATMENTS: PHYSICAL AND SURGICAL MANIPULATIONS

Surgical Spinal Cord Relaxation (Cervicolordodesis)

Description: Surgical procedure to fix the cervical spine (in the neck) to restrict forward bending.

Rationale: It is suggested that the hard MS scar in parts of the spine subject to extreme motion, e.g., the neck, tends to restrict the normal "viscoelastic flow" of the tissue, i.e., its free movement, and to bring abnormal pressure to bear on nerve fibers in this part of the cord. Surgical restriction of neck movement would prevent this.

Evaluation: This procedure is alleged to be helpful in MS, but no data have been provided.

Risks/Costs: Both high.

Conclusion: This therapy is without value in MS.

In the opinion of the Committee, there appears to be no generally accepted scientific basis for use of this therapy. It has never been tested in a proper controlled trial. Its use carries significant risk. It is very expensive.

MISCELLANEOUS EMPIRICAL TREATMENTS: PHYSICAL AND SURGICAL MANIPULATIONS

Vertebral Artery Surgery

Description: An operation devised to eliminate kinking or narrowing of the vertebral arteries in the neck.

Rationale: The two vertebral arteries take their origin low in the neck and pass upward and backward, entering the skull along with the spinal cord. On the underside of the brainstem they join to form the basilar artery. The vertebral-basilar artery system provides most or all of the blood supply to the brainstem, cerebellum, and part of the cerebrum.

It has been proposed that "congenital or acquired partial extraluminal obstruction of the proximal vertebral artery initially impedes blood flow and, after a period of time, converts into a functional stenosis" (narrowing). "Slowly progressive degeneration of the myelin sheaths of the nerve fibers in the brainstem can result from chronic ischemic hypoxia" (lack of oxygen owing to impaired blood flow).

Evaluation: Nine MS patients who had signs and symptoms compatible with involvement in the vertebral-basilar artery distribution had operations performed "to correct the partial extraluminal obstruction of their proximal vertebral arteries between July 9, 1976, and February 28, 1978." At the time of the report all nine patients "experienced partial restoration of lost neurologic function."

The report does not include specific information concerning the diagnosis and state of the disease in most of the patients, nor is there any quantification of changes between pre- and postoperative status. The period of postoperative observation is not stated, but the report was published the same year as some of the operations. There were no controls.

A number of considerations produce serious doubts concerning such surgery for MS. The lesions of MS are not limited to the vertebral-basilar system. Numerous attempts to enhance blood flow to the nervous system by other means have failed to alter the course of MS, and many such agents and procedures have been generally discarded as ineffective.

A variant of this approach, in use in a limited area of Great Britain, is the surgical production of an arteriovenous fistula (an artificial connection between an artery and a vein, bypassing the capillary bed) at a peripheral site, such as the foot, presumed to alter blood flow in the CNS.

Risks/Costs: The risks and costs of surgery and of hospitalization.

Conclusion: The existing evidence does not support the conclusion that these procedures may be effective in the treatment of MS.

In the opinion of the Committee, there appears to be no generally accepted scientific basis for use of this therapy. It has never been tested in a proper controlled trial. Its use carries significant risk. It is very expensive.

MISCELLANEOUS EMPIRICAL TREATMENTS: PHYSICAL AND SURGICAL MANIPULATIONS

Ultrasound

Description: Repeated application of ultrasound, i.e., high frequency sound, to the area of the back next to the spinal column (backbone).

Rationale: Ultrasound has great value as a diagnostic tool, which permits doctors to probe certain parts of the body without harming the area probed. It is sometimes used to reduce pain and spasm in muscles. In patients with MS, it is claimed that ultrasound "treatment" promotes the flow of lymph in lymph vessels draining the spinal cord, and thus affects the disease process.

Evaluation: Use of ultrasound in MS has been stressed by certain clinics in Austria in the last few years. No controlled studies have been published, and reports of its effectiveness reflect mainly clinical impressions rather than objective observations. It is unclear how a treatment directed to the spinal cord could affect lesions in the brain. As noted earlier, a variety of treatments directed to improving blood and lymph flow in the CNS have been tried over many years and judged ineffective.

Risks/Costs: Cost of repeated treatment is high.

Conclusion: The evidence suggests that this treatment is unlikely to be effective in MS. The high price clearly reflects commercial exploitation.

In the opinion of the Committee, there appears to be no generally accepted scientific basis for use of this therapy. It has never been tested in a proper controlled trial. Risks are undetermined. It is very expensive.

MISCELLANEOUS EMPIRICAL TREATMENTS: PHYSICAL AND SURGICAL MANIPULATIONS

Magnetotherapy

Description: Repeated application of a low-frequency pulsing magnetic field. The strength of the field and the duration and frequency of exposure can be varied. Fifteen daily exposures at 2–10 H and less than 50×10^{-4} T are recommended.

Rationale: Among many theories, a pulsing magnetic field is thought to improve cell functions, circulation, and oxygenation and to reduce edema, inflammation, and scarring. Perhaps more significant, it acts as the equivalent of repetitive high-frequency electrical stimulation of nerve fibers exposed to the field.

Evaluation: Alleged to be of value in MS, as well as a large variety of other illnesses. A controlled clinical trial of magnetotherapy has been carried out in one center in Hungary. Nine of 10 patients with chronic stabilized disease showed mild to moderate improvement in spasticity (and accompanying pain) and half were reported to show improvement in cerebellar and bladder functions, whereas only 2 of 10 patients given a placebo exposure improved. Improvement was maintained over 4–16 weeks, with a slow return to pretreatment status. Reexposure resulted again in improvement. The treatment was effective, when applied to the earlier placebo group, in 8 of 10 cases. Results in an uncontrolled open study of 104 patients agreed with those obtained in the controlled study.

Risks/Costs: Unknown.

Conclusion: This treatment is not yet proven. Further controlled observations are awaited with interest.

In the opinion of the Committee, there appears to be no generally accepted scientific basis for use of this therapy. It has never been tested in a proper controlled trial. Risks are undetermined.

MISCELLANEOUS EMPIRICAL TREATMENTS: PHYSICAL AND SURGICAL MANIPULATIONS

Dental Occlusal Therapy

Description: Correction of dental malocclusion with occlusal splints and other procedures, attention to other dental needs, and physical therapy to the muscles and structures of the temporomandibular joints. (A diet low in animal fat, with increased oil intake, vitamin and mineral supplements, and avoidance of refined foods [especially sugars] are also recommended.)

Rationale: Dental malocclusions may be associated with dental distress, especially in the muscles and structures of the temporomandibular joints, and supposedly with decreased stress resistance in certain systemic muscle groups. The affected joints and muscles produce a continuing sensory input to the brain, which is thought to result in decreased neurologic output and demyelination.

Evaluation: It is claimed that correction of occlusal dysfunction will improve about 70% of the systemic musculature that shows lowered stress resistance in MS patients. Any specific muscle may be expected to show about a 30% improvement. There is no known scientific basis for the claim that alterations in sensory input can affect the integrity of myelin. The degree of clinical improvement said to be observed can be accounted for easily as: (a) subjective; (b) placebo effects; (c) muscle dysfunction due to malocclusion being inaccurately diagnosed as MS. It is improbable that dental distress is a significant contributing variable in the MS disease development process.

Risks/Costs: Information concerning risks and costs was not reported.

Conclusion: Review of the literature suggests that there is neither a scientific basis nor acceptable medical evidence that the therapeutic program described could favorably influence the MS disease process.

In the opinion of the Committee, there appears to be no generally accepted scientific basis for use of this therapy. It has never been tested in a proper controlled trial. It is relatively free of serious adverse side-effects during long-term use. It is very expensive.

MISCELLANEOUS EMPIRICAL TREATMENTS: PHYSICAL AND SURGICAL MANIPULATIONS

Replacement of Mercury Amalgam Fillings

Description: Removal and replacement of all fillings made of silver and mercury amalgam.

Rationale: This procedure or even the removal of filled teeth is based on the unsubstantiated claim that mercury leaks from amalgam fillings and damages the immune system, thus causing a broad range of problems, said to include MS and leukemia. "Are your silver fillings poisoning you?" One dentist has developed a "mercury sensitivity test." Another theory suggests that the leaking mercury combines with nerve in the root canal and induces autoimmunization.

Evaluation: There is no sound epidemiologic evidence to relate MS to dental work. The procedures described are carried out by dentists in the absence of medical consultation and are quite lucrative.

Risks/Costs: Harmless but quite expensive.

Conclusion: There is no evidence to suggest that this procedure is of value in MS.

In the opinion of the Committee, there appears to be no generally accepted scientific basis for use of this therapy. It has never been tested in a proper controlled trial. It is relatively free of serious adverse side-effects during long-term use. It is very expensive.

MISCELLANEOUS EMPIRICAL TREATMENTS: PHYSICAL AND SURGICAL MANIPULATIONS

Implantation of Brain

Description: Surgical implantation of pig brain in the abdominal wall.

Rationale: Unclear.

Evaluation: Implantation of foreign tissue (as in cellular therapy) is a recurring theme in medicine. The newest variation on this theme is implantation of pig brain in MS patients. According to newspaper accounts, 13 of 15 patients reported symptomatic improvement within 24 h. A critique by the German MS Society pointed out the absence of a scientific rationale for this procedure and its many dangers. The claimed results are regarded as a placebo effect.

Risks/Costs: The procedure is expensive ($200), and carries the usual risks of surgery, in particular infection and abscess formation at the implantation site, where the pig tissue undergoes rejection as a foreign graft. Such brain grafts also carry the risk of inducing autoimmune brain disease resembling the animal model EAE or transmitting pig viruses to the "treated" patient. By February 1982, two of 38 MS patients treated with this procedure in Germany had developed severe complications and one had died.

Conclusion: The evidence examined demonstrates that this treatment should be regarded as ineffective and dangerous.

In the opinion of the Committee, this therapy should not be used because of reported harmful effects.

MISCELLANEOUS EMPIRICAL TREATMENTS: PHYSICAL AND SURGICAL MANIPULATIONS

Hysterectomy

Description: Surgical removal of the uterus.

Rationale: It is suggested that progesterone can induce autoimmunization. It is then said to form immune complexes with antiprogesterone antibody, and these can damage various targeted tissues, among them the central and peripheral nervous systems. The lesions may manifest edema, inflammation, and tissue necrosis. In the CNS, they may mimic MS.

Evaluation: Alleged to benefit MS. No data are provided to support this claim.

Risks/Costs: Risk is that of major surgery. Cost is high.

Conclusion: This procedure is not recommended for MS.

In the opinion of the Committee, there appears to be no generally accepted scientific basis for use of this therapy. It has never been tested in a proper controlled trial. It is very expensive.

MISCELLANEOUS EMPIRICAL TREATMENTS: DIET

Allergen-Free Diet

Description: Regular use of a diet from which foods are eliminated that are known to produce hives, other skin eruptions, asthmatic attacks, etc.

Rationale: This diet is based on the theory that the lesions of MS might be some sort of allergic reaction to common allergens from the environment.

Evaluation: The theory that MS might be allergic in character had its adherents in the late 1940s and early 1950s. One of the first diets recommended for MS was an allergen-free diet. Such a diet may be effective in treating diseases that are allergic in origin, notably hives, certain skin eruptions, hay fever, asthmatic attacks, etc. The use of allergen-free diets in MS has been largely dropped from physicians' practices today.

Risks/Costs: Short-term use of the allergen-free diet has no associated risk.

Conclusion: It is not known if this diet is effective. The necessary controlled studies have not been done.

In the opinion of the Committee, there appears to be no generally accepted scientific basis for use of this therapy. It has never been tested in a proper controlled trial. It is relatively free of serious adverse side-effects during long-term use.

MISCELLANEOUS EMPIRICAL TREATMENTS: DIET

Gluten-Free Diet

Description: A balanced diet excluding wheat and rye.

Rationale: The prevalence of MS is high in areas of the world that raise and consume wheat and rye, which are gluten-containing grains, and low in areas that consume rice and corn, which do not contain gluten.

Evaluation: A balanced diet excluding wheat and rye was suggested for use by MS patients. Subsequently, a diet was publicized that eliminated gluten and restricted carbohydrates, coffee, and alcohol. A 2-year uncontrolled study of a gluten-free diet reported that both relapses and progression occurred in patients on the diet. However, the number of relapses and degree of progression could be readily explained by the natural course of MS. A small double-blind study (28 patients) showed no evidence of benefit from use of the diet.

Risks/Costs: Elimination of wheat and rye from the diet may result in inadequate protein intake, unless protein is provided from other sources.

Conclusion: On the basis of the available data, this diet must be considered ineffective in MS.

In the opinion of the Committee, there appears to be no generally accepted scientific basis for use of this therapy. It has never been tested in a proper controlled trial. It is relatively free of serious adverse side-effects during long-term use.

MISCELLANEOUS EMPIRICAL TREATMENTS: DIET

Raw Food, Evers Diet

Description: A diet containing only natural (unprocessed) foods, including a daily intake of germinated wheat.

Rationale: A German physician, Dr. Joseph Evers, believed that many illnesses were due to unnatural methods of production and processing of foods. His diet recommended the use of raw root vegetables, whole wheat bread, cheese, raw milk, raw eggs, butter, honey, and raw ham. Natural wine and brandy were permitted. Salt, sugar, confections, and condiments were forbidden. Also forbidden were leafy greens, stalks, and certain vegetables (salads, rhubarb, asparagus, cauliflower).

Evaluation: Although the Evers diet has been used by some patients with MS, there is no evidence from the results that it affects the natural course of the disease. There also would seem to be no scientific basis for the claim that processed foods are chemically different from natural foods. None of the common food additives has been shown to produce lesions resembling those of MS.

Risks/Costs: There are no significant risks. Many so-called natural foods are expensive.

Conclusion: On the basis of existing information, it appears that this diet should be considered ineffective in MS.

In the opinion of the Committee, there appears to be no generally accepted scientific basis for use of this therapy. It has never been tested in a proper controlled trial. It is relatively free of serious adverse side-effects during long-term use.

MISCELLANEOUS EMPIRICAL TREATMENTS: DIET

MacDougal Diet

Description: This diet combines a low-fat diet with a gluten-free diet and adds supplements of vitamins and minerals.

Rationale: The proponent of the diet, Professor Roger Mac-Dougal, a writer and dramatist, believed that the combination diet was responsible for the almost complete disappearance of his symptoms of MS.

Evaluation: There has been no scientific evidence that the MacDougal diet affects the natural course of MS.

Risks/Costs: Risks are negligible.

Conclusion: There appears to be no scientific evidence that this diet is effective in MS.

In the opinion of the Committee, there appears to be no generally accepted scientific basis for use of this therapy. It has never been tested in a proper controlled trial. It is relatively free of serious adverse side-effects during long-term use.

Pectin- and Fructose-Restricted Diet (Based on Methanol Hypothesis)

Description: A diet from which unripe fruits, fruit juices, and pectin-containing fruits and vegetables are eliminated, supplemented with menadione (vitamin K_3).

Rationale: A treatment based on the hypothesis that methanol (wood alcohol) produced by metabolism of pectins (complex sugars) is converted to formaldehyde, which can bind to myelin components and lead to autoimmunization and consequent tissue damage. This process is thought to be exaggerated by ingestion of sugars containing fructose, which is said to block the breakdown of formaldehyde, and pectins, which may contain some methanol. Menadione promotes the formation of tissue components (sphingomyelin), which may antagonize the methanol effect.

Evaluation: In a sizeable uncontrolled series of patients on this diet, followed for more than a year, relapses and exacerbations occurred, and a significant number of patients deteriorated while on the diet. About one-third of the patients dropped out of the trial. In the absence of controls, it is impossible to judge whether there was some reduction in progression or attacks. However, the results were similar to those obtained with other unproven therapies.

Risks/Costs: It is difficult and time-consuming to instruct patients in the use of the diet.

Conclusion: The methanol hypothesis and the dietary regimen based on it remain unproven.

In the opinion of the Committee, there appears to be no generally accepted scientific basis for use of this therapy. It has never been tested in a proper controlled trial. It is relatively free of serious adverse side-effects during long-term use.

MISCELLANEOUS EMPIRICAL TREATMENTS: DIET

"Cambridge" and Other Liquid Diets

Description: A balanced, very low calorie liquid, used in treatment of obesity. Calorie intake is 330/day with a suboptimal level of protein at 22 g/day. Extra potassium is supplied.

Rationale: Studies have shown no acceptable rationale for use of this diet in MS, except to correct obesity.

Risk/Costs: Intense crash diets may lead to potassium deficiency, and several cases of sudden death resulting from such deficiency have been reported. The diet should only be undertaken with medical or other professional supervision.

Conclusion: Based on the evidence examined, this diet is not recommended for treatment of MS.

In the opinion of the Committee, there appears to be no generally accepted scientific basis for use of this therapy. It has never been tested in a proper controlled trial. Its use carries significant risk.

MISCELLANEOUS EMPIRICAL TREATMENTS: DIET

Sucrose- and Tobacco-Free Diet

Description: Elimination of all food products containing sucrose in the form of cane, brown, or maple sugars, molasses, sorghum, or dates; also products containing propylene glycol or glycol stearate (in shampoos). Tobacco is not to be used in any form.

Rationale: The diet is based on the belief that MS is caused by a form of allergy to sucrose or tobacco, as well as to the food additive propylene glycol. Glycol distearate, a constituent of many shampoos, is also incriminated.

Evaluation: The recommendation is based on personal experiences of eight MS patients with elimination diets of the type recommended. The diet is said to be ineffective in patients older than 50 years of age. No controlled study has been carried out.

Risks/Costs: The use of substitute sweeteners may be expensive.

Conclusion: This therapy remains unproven.

In the opinion of the Committee, there appears to be no generally accepted scientific basis for use of this therapy. It has never been tested in a proper controlled trial. It is relatively free of serious adverse side-effects during long-term use.

MISCELLANEOUS EMPIRICAL TREATMENTS: DIET

Vitamins

Description: Individual vitamins or combinations of vitamins are taken in capsule or liquid form, as a supplement to a normal diet.

Rationale: It is assumed that MS may result from an unidentified vitamin deficiency.

Evaluation: Beginning in the late 1920s and continuing into the 1960s there have been reports in the scientific literature of vitamins in the treatment of MS. Various vitamins have been used alone or in a variety of combinations. Vitamins have been given orally (by mouth), parenterally (by injection), and intraspinally. Vitamin preparations used have included: thiamine (B_1), nicotinic acid (niacin), vitamin B_{12}, ascorbic acid (vitamin C), tocopherol (vitamin E), and liver therapy. Specific combinations of vitamins used have included fat-soluble vitamins (A, D, E, and K) with ammonium chloride, thiamine, and nicotinic acid. Improvement has been reported to occur in from 0% of patients in some studies up to 100% in other studies. None of the studies was subjected to the criteria and controls now used in the scientific evaluation of therapies for MS.

Risks/Costs: There is no evidence in animal experiments that vitamin deficiency can produce lesions resembling those of MS. Vitamins A and D in high doses are toxic. Supplementation with vitamins adds significantly to the cost of a normal balanced diet.

Conclusion: Adequate intake of vitamins is advised in all patients with MS, but there appears to be no scientific proof that supplementary doses of vitamins, alone or in combination, favorably affect the course of the disease.

In the opinion of the Committee, there appears to be no generally accepted scientific basis for use of this therapy. It has never been tested in a proper controlled trial. Long-term use may be associated with significant serious side-effects.

MISCELLANEOUS EMPIRICAL TREATMENTS: DIET

Megavitamin Therapy

Description: Massive doses of vitamins.

Rationale: As with other vitamin supplementation, large doses are used to make up for a presumed deficiency in uptake or utilization of one or more vitamins.

Evaluation: Megavitamin therapy has recently received widespread publicity, especially in Canada and in a few localities in the United States. Massive doses of vitamins have been said to be effective in the treatment of MS. "These reports are based usually on individual testimonials, and the Multiple Sclerosis Society of Canada must affirm that there is still no reliable scientific evidence to indicate that megavitamin therapy in any way influences the course of the disease."

Risks/Costs: It should be noted that excessive doses of some vitamins, especially A and D, may produce toxic effects. When pyridoxine (vitamin B_6) is used in high doses, it sometimes produces disease of the peripheral nervous system, with weakness and loss of balance. This is especially a problem in patients who are already weak. Vitamins are expensive.

Conclusion: There appears to be no reliable evidence that megavitamin therapy influences the course of MS.

In the opinion of the Committee, there appears to be no generally accepted scientific basis for use of this therapy. It has never been tested in a proper controlled trial. Long-term use may be associated with significant serious side-effects.

MISCELLANEOUS EMPIRICAL TREATMENTS: DIET

Megascorbic Therapy

Description: Massive doses of vitamin C (ascorbic acid), referred to as an "orthomolecular" treatment.

Rationale: The claim is made that many people have a defective gene governing liver enzymes concerned with carbohydrate metabolism. The consequent defect in vitamin C production, identified by a failure of spillover of this vitamin in the urine, results in "hypoascorbemia" and "chronic subclinical scurvy." This in turn is considered to underlie MS as well as a variety of other diseases, among them cancer, heart disease, stroke, arthritis, leukemia, diabetes, infectious diseases, "and many others." In the case of MS, high vitamin C levels are said to promote the patient's ability to produce IFN and resist viral infection.

Evaluation: The many diseases for which this therapy is proposed are unrelated to each other and none has any known relation to vitamin C. The Committee believes no scientifically adequate trial of this vitamin at megadose levels in MS has ever been carried out.

Risks/Costs: Continued treatment with vitamin C at the suggested levels is very expensive. Medical evidence has shown that high levels of ascorbic acid intake can produce stomach problems and kidney stones.

Conclusion: The value of megascorbic therapy in MS is unproven and this treatment, therefore, is not recommended.

In the opinion of the Committee, there appears to be no generally accepted scientific basis for use of this therapy. It has never been tested in a proper controlled trial. Its use carries significant risk.

MISCELLANEOUS EMPIRICAL TREATMENTS: DIET

Minerals

Description: Addition of various mineral salts to diet.

Rationale: These, in almost all cases, were empirical attempts to use agents found helpful to the general state of well-being in other diseases.

Evaluation: In the 1880s, associates of the French neurologist Charcot reported the use of zinc phosphates in the treatment of MS. Among the early therapies for MS, prior to 1935, were included other minerals, such as potassium bromide or iodide, antimony, gold, silver, mercury, arsenic, thorium, and metallic salts. In modern times, essential minerals have been combined with vitamin supplements in a program of supplying added nutrients. There do not seem to be recent reports in the scientific literature on use of minerals alone as a specific treatment for MS. It was reported recently that there is a deficiency of manganese in MS. This led to the recommendation that buckwheat cakes, an excellent source of manganese, be included regularly in the diet of MS patients. No results have been reported. Zinc has also been proposed as a possibly effective treatment for MS, but there have been no reports of controlled studies. Another recent suggestion is long-continued ingestion of potassium, in the form of potassium gluconate.

Risks/Costs: Many minerals are toxic when ingested at any level above the traces found in normal foods.

Conclusion: There appears to be no clear evidence that any of these regimens should be considered effective in MS.

In the opinion of the Committee, there appears to be no generally accepted scientific basis for use of this therapy. It has never been tested in a proper controlled trial. Risks are undetermined.

Cerebrosides

Description: Dietary supplementation with fatty acids of cerebrosides from beef spinal cord.

Rationale: Long-chain fatty acids rapidly increase in the brain during myelination in infancy. It was suggested that dietary deficiency in such fatty acids might play a role in MS.

Evaluation: Fatty acids prepared from cerebrosides derived from beef spinal cord were fed for 18 months to patients with MS. One sizeable scientific study with matched experimental and placebo control groups demonstrated that the experimental group did not fare any better than the control.

Risks/Costs: Negligible.

Conclusion: On the basis of published evidence, this treatment is considered ineffective in MS.

In the opinion of the Committee, there appears to be no generally accepted scientific basis for use of this therapy. It has never been tested in a proper controlled trial. It is relatively free of serious adverse side-effects during long-term use.

MISCELLANEOUS EMPIRICAL TREATMENTS: DIET

Aloe Vera

Description: Juice of the *Aloe vera* plant, available over the counter, taken by mouth on a regular basis.

Rationale: Aloe vera juice contains vitamins, amino acids, and minerals and doubtless can serve as a valuable food supplement. The promotional literature for the product, however, also asserts it will cure a wide variety of unrelated conditions, and claims that the juice is antibacterial and antiinflammatory.

Evaluation: Aloe vera juice has been taken by a number of patients with MS: Anecdotal reports are available of patients who recovered from an acute attack of MS after taking the juice repeatedly. This would appear to reflect the natural history of the disease and not real therapeutic effect. There have been no controlled trials of this material. The FDA states that: "There is no scientific evidence to support allegations that *Aloe vera* is effective as a treatment for cancer, diabetes, or any other serious disease."

Aloe vera has also been combined with other substances in a program marketed as "Herbalife." Individual patients have been reported to show favorable responses.

Risks/Costs: The juice is not generally harmful, but it can produce mild diarrhea and skin hypersensitivity.

Conclusion: Aloe vera is not recommended for use in MS.

In the opinion of the Committee, there appears to be no generally accepted scientific basis for use of this therapy. It has never been tested in a proper controlled trial. Risks are undetermined.

MISCELLANEOUS EMPIRICAL TREATMENTS: DIET

Enzymes

Description: A diet similar to the Evers diet (natural or unprocessed foods, also low fat), supplemented with plant and bacterial enzymes (Wobenzym), normal digestive enzymes, vitamins, and minerals (Vitafestal), lipolytic enzymes (Bilicomb), and others (Panpur, Panzynorm).

Rationale: A Swiss physician, Dr. F. Schmid, has recommended a wide spectrum of enzyme substitution at mealtimes, "as long as the causal enzyme defects are not known for individual degeneration diseases." He suggests that enzyme preparations "supplement the natural supply of the foodstuffs and act as replacements in cases where a consistent diet with undenatured foodstuffs cannot be implemented."

Evaluation: There is no convincing evidence that patients with MS have any defect in digestive function. The rationale provided does not, in fact, claim that such evidence exists. The enzyme supplement is, nevertheless, recommended by its proponent for MS and other completely unrelated diseases of the nervous system that are not known to share a common dietary mechanism. No controlled studies of such supplementation have ever been done.

Risks/Costs: Purchase of the recommended supplements adds significantly to the cost of a normal diet.

Conclusion: Enzyme supplementation is not recommended.

In the opinion of the Committee, there appears to be no generally accepted scientific basis for use of this therapy. It has never been tested in a proper controlled trial. It is relatively free of serious adverse side-effects during long-term use.

Selected Bibliography

Brown JR (1980). Problems in evaluating new treatments for multiple sclerosis. *Neurology* 30 (Part II):8–11.

Hommes OR, ed. (1986). *Multiple Sclerosis Research in Europe*. Boston: MTP Press.

Matthews WB, Acheson ED, Batchelor JR, Weller RO (1985). *McAlpine's Multiple Sclerosis*. Edinburgh: Churchill-Livingstone.

McDonald WI, D. Silberberg (1986). *Multiple Sclerosis*. London: Butterworths.

Rudick RA, Herndon RM, eds. (1985). *Disorders of Myelin*. New York: Thieme-Stratton, pp. 85–196. (Seminars in neurology, vol. 5.)

Schapiro RT (1987). *Symptom Management in Multiple Sclerosis*. New York: Demos Publications.

Scheinberg LC, Holland NJ, eds. (1987). *Multiple Sclerosis: A Guide for Patients and Their Families*, 2nd ed. New York: Raven Press.

Sibley WA (1988). Risk factors in multiple sclerosis. In: Serlupi Crescenzi G, ed. *A Multidisciplinary Approach to Myelin Diseases*. New York: Plenum Press. (NATO Advanced Research Series.)

Smith CR, Aisen ML, Scheinberg L (1986). Symptomatic management of multiple sclerosis. In: McDonald WI, Silberberg D, eds. *Multiple Sclerosis*. London: Butterworths.

Waksman BH, Reingold SC, Reynolds WE (1988). *Research on Multiple Sclerosis*. New York: Demos Publications.

For a more detailed account of older methods of treatment:

Sibley WA (1970). Drug treatment of multiple sclerosis. In: Vinken P, Bruyn GW, eds. *Handbook of Clinical Neurology*, vol. 9, Ch. 12. New York: American Elsevier; Amsterdam: North Holland.

Hyperbaric oxygen, 159–160
Hyperimmune colostrum, 150–151
Hyperreflexia, 7
Hysterectomy, 174

Ibuprofen, 37
IFMSS, 14,124
Imipramine for urinary frequency, 99
Immune system, 50–52
  and causes of MS, 11–12
  treatment, 25–26
Immunobiological revitalization, 144
Immunoglobulins, 142–143
Immunomodulators, 48,72–79
Immunosuppression, 33,49,61–71
Imuran. *See* Azathioprine
Incoordination, treatment, 95–96,103
Indocin, 37
Indomethacin, 32,37
Infections
  encephalomyelitis following, 50,81
  treatment, 24
Inflammation, treatment, 24–25
Influenza virus, 88,117
INH (isoniazid), 26,96
Injected treatments for MS, 125–149
Inosiplix, 87
Interferon
  -α, 24,48,49,83–84,86
  -β, 24,48,49,83–84,86
  -γ, 12,24,48,51,83,85,86,139
International Federation of Multiple Sclerosis Societies (IFMSS), 14,124
Intraglobin, 142
Inuit (Eskimos), 10,121
Isoniazid (INH), 26,96
Isonicotinic acid hydrazide

(INH), 26,96
Isoprinosine, 87
Isopropamide for urinary frequency, 99

Ketazolam for spasticity, 109
Ketoprofen, 37
Kurtzke scale, 13,15–16,138

Le Gac therapy, 154
Leukemia, 68,184
Leukeran, 69
Levamisole, 48,72
Lioresal. *See* Baclofen for spasticity
Lomustine, 70
Long-term management and rehabilitation, 103–104
Low-fat diet, 103–122,170,178
Lymphocytapheresis (leukapheresis), 48–49,67
Lymphocytes
  B-cells, 51,52
  T-cells, 50–52,60,75,77,83
    helper, 47,51,52,57,72,73
    killer, 51,57
    suppressor, 51,52,72–73,79
  transfer, 79
Lymphokines, 51
Lymphoma, non-Hodgkin's, 53

MacDougal diet, 26,178
Macroglia, 1,3
Macrophages, 51
Magnesium, 147
Magnetic resonance imaging (MRI), 6,8,9,16,20,44,159
  cf. CT scan, 6,8,9
Magnetotherapy, 169
Major histocompatibility complex, 60; *see also* HLA
Manganese, 185
Mannitol, 44
Marijuana for spasticity, 112
Megascorbic therapy, 184
Megavitamin therapy, 183
Menadione, 179

6-Mercaptopurine, 68
Mercury amalgam fillings, re-
placement, 172
Metabolic disturbance, treat-
ment, 20–22
Metabolic therapy, 152
Metamucil, 100
Methanol hypothesis, 179
Methisoprinol, 50,87
Methotrexate, 68
Methylprednisolone, 25,27–
28,31–34
intrathecal, 35
Mimicry, molecular, 12
Minerals, dietary, 185
Minimal Record of Disability,
14
Mitoxantrone, 71
Molecular mimicry, 12
Monoamine oxidase inhibitors,
97,101
Monoclonal antibodies, antilymphocyte, 60–61
Morphine for spasticity, 95
Motor disturbance, treatment,
93–96
Motrin, 37
Multiple sclerosis (MS)
causes, 11–12
course of, without treatment,
12–13
definition, 4
diagnosis, 4–10
electrodiagnostic tests, 8
neurological examination,
6,7
spinal fluid changes, 6–7,9
epidemiology, 10–11
sex, 11
map of principal lesions, 2
progress of, measurement,
13–16
symptoms, 5–6
see also Treatment of MS en-
tries
Myasthenia gravis, 77

Myelin, 2–4,14,130,147,170
Myelin basic protein, 25
treatment with, 49,50,80,81

Nalfon, 37
Naprosyn, 37
Naproxen, 37
Natural killer cells, 83
Nerve cells, 1
Nerve fiber (axon), 1–4,14
Nerve stimulation, transcuta-
neous, 161
Nervous system irradiation, 43
Neurological examination, 6,7
Nicotinic acid, 182
Nifedipine, 116
Non-Hodgkin's lymphoma, 53
Nonsteroidal antiinflammatory
drugs (NSAIDs), 32,37,96
Novatrone, 71
Nystatin, 25,155

Occupational therapy, 95
Octacosanol, 130,152
Oligodendroglia, 1,2
Orgosein, 131–132
Orgotein, 131,132
Orthomolecular treatment, 184
Orudis, 37
Oxybutyrin for urinary fre-
quency, 99
Oxygen radicals, 40,131

Pain, treatment, 96–97
Palosein, 131–132
Pancorphen, 127
Pancreatic extract (Depropa-
nex), 126
Pancreatin, 145
Panpur, 188
Panzynorm, 188
Parkinsonism, 88, 117
Paroxysmal symptoms, 103
Pectin- and fructose-restricted
diet, 179
Pemoline, 98, 118
D-Penicillamine, 42